The Power of Protest in Healthcare

of related interest

Minority Ethnic Voices in Healthcare Professions
Strategies for Career Empowerment and Creating Inclusive Settings
Heena Mahmood
ISBN 978 1 80501 154 5
eISBN 978 1 80501 155 2

Health Equality and Social Justice in Old Age
A Frontline Perspective
Dr Riaz Dharamshi
ISBN 978 1 83997 365 9
eISBN 978 1 83997 381 9

Occupational Therapy, Disability Activism, and Me
Challenging Ableism in Healthcare
Georgia Vine
ISBN 978 1 83997 667 4
eISBN 978 1 83997 668 1

Occupational Therapy Disruptors
What Global OT Practice Can Teach Us About Innovation, Culture, and Community
Sheela Roy Ivlev
Foreword by Juman Simaan
ISBN 978 1 83997 665 0
eISBN 978 1 83997 666 7

THE POWER OF PROTEST IN HEALTHCARE

Lessons From a Doctor's Journey to Activism

DR MEENAL VIZ

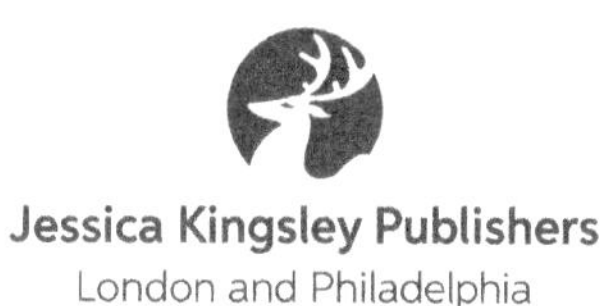

Jessica Kingsley Publishers
London and Philadelphia

First published in Great Britain in 2026 by Jessica Kingsley Publishers
An imprint of John Murray Press

1

Front cover image source: Shutterstock®.

A CIP catalogue record for this title is available from the British Library and the Library of Congress

ISBN 978 1 83997 841 8
eISBN 978 1 83997 842 5

Printed and bound in Great Britain by Clays Ltd

Jessica Kingsley Publishers' policy is to use papers that are natural, renewable and recyclable products and made from wood grown in sustainable forests. The logging and manufacturing processes are expected to conform to the environmental regulations of the country of origin.

Jessica Kingsley Publishers
Carmelite House
50 Victoria Embankment
London EC4Y 0DZ

www.jkp.com

John Murray Press
Part of Hodder & Stoughton Ltd
An Hachette Company

The authorised representative in the EEA is Hachette Ireland, 8 Castlecourt Centre, Castleknock Road, Castleknock, Dublin 15, D15 YF6A, Ireland (email: info@hbgi.ie)

Contents

Preface

A Letter to My Daughters

My dearest Radhika, Anoushka and Shivika,

When I look at you all, I see a future where you've reached heights no other woman in our family has ever reached.

I see a future where you're not treated differently because of the colour of your skin.

I see a world where you don't carry the weight of generational trauma our family has inherited over the years.

I know that this is a world that is still all too far away, but I am committed to do everything in my power to make it a reality.

I know that I can't change the world overnight, but I can start by changing the world around you.

As you grow older, I will pass the baton to you.

By then, I hope there is little work left to be done.

My life is dedicated to you, my three girls.

I love you all with every fibre of my being.

* * *

This book is dedicated to you, Radhika, Anoushka and

Shivika. I hope it acts as a catalyst to ignite your spark in finding your voice and speaking your truth. I want you to bloom, not just with beauty, but with a purpose that extends beyond yourselves.

I am sure you will all learn about the Covid-19 pandemic through your history lessons in school. Who knows what sort of internet world we will be living in over the next few years; you might even have robots teaching you at school!

There are many harsh truths about the pandemic which cannot be swept away; they must be documented and the truth must be told. Anything less would be an injustice to all the families who lost their loved ones to the deadly virus. Information spreads fast these days, and by the time you read this book, I am certain there will be a plethora of accounts describing what happened during this global health crisis.

I hope that, as adults, you use my experience and my learnings from this book to advocate for yourself when you feel that you are faced with any form of injustice.

I want you all to be the beacons of hope for those who need you the most and for those who feel they may not have the agency to speak up.

* * *

Radhika, you are my firstborn, and you gave me the greatest privilege of becoming a mother. I still remember the moment we found out we were having a girl and I immediately looked at your father and said, 'We will name her Radhika. Seeker of justice.' This was back in January 2020, when we felt that nothing could ever harm our family. The happy bubble we'd built soon shimmered with a new kind of fear, a virus lurking on the horizon, a shadow threatening our sunshine.

I was on a cocktail of medicines to ease my pregnancy sickness with you. Everyone told me that it was a good sign – a sign that you were growing. But through the haze, there was a glimmer. Each sip of unappealing tea, each bland bite of biscuit, was a tiny victory.

Despite these minor inconveniences, I was grateful to experience everything that came with being pregnant. Your father would take me for long evening drives to distract me from my sickness and we would sit in the McDonald's car park sharing an ice-cream and discussing cute nicknames for you. 'We'll call her Radhi Boo Boo and we'll continue to call her that until she gets embarrassed in front of her friends.' Your father had everything planned – your first day at school, your first tennis racket – and he had even gone as far as thinking about how he could be the coolest, yet most embarrassing dad any girl could have. He even planned how he would split his time between all his children when they were grown up.

Radhika and Anoushka, neither of you was in existence and your father had already dedicated his life's plan to you both.

During the early stages of the pandemic, we had faith that we would be protected from the virus. After all, we were living in a country with the world's greatest academics sitting in parliament and making the key decisions to protect the nation. But the virus insidiously crept up on us, and doctors across the country were getting infected. The height of suffering we were subjected to in the hospital was unfathomable. No amount of medical training could prepare us for what we experienced.

Overnight, we went from discussing cute nicknames for you, Radhika, to mapping out our emergency birthing plans in case I had to deliver you at home.

As the pandemic unfolded, the world witnessed a spectrum of human responses – from acts of selfless heroism to deplorable displays of selfishness. Healthcare workers, the frontline warriors against the virus, risked their own lives to care for the sick, often working under immense pressure and facing shortages of protective equipment. Ordinary citizens stepped up to volunteer, providing support to the vulnerable and helping to maintain essential services.

Amid the chaos, there were also those who exploited the pandemic for personal gain, hoarding supplies, spreading misinformation and engaging in profiteering. The virus, it seemed, had the uncanny ability to amplify both the best and worst aspects of human nature.

Your father is the most honest, selfless and hardworking man I know. He would volunteer to help his department with the sick and suspected Covid-19 patients just to make sure his colleagues wouldn't get infected. Whispers of equipment shortages turned to frustrated shouts, only to be met with a chilling silence. Doctors, once vocal advocates for their patients, were being muzzled. It was a betrayal that gnawed at him, a stark contrast to the oath he swore to uphold. He saw the fear in their eyes, not just of the virus, but of the truth they were forbidden to speak.

Your father was way ahead of all the headlines and news. He would spend his evenings after work reading all the latest research papers on the virus. I remember watching him fall asleep on the sofa with his laptop on his chest, purely from exhaustion. Back then, I mistook his exhaustion for the burden of long hours. Now, I see it for what it truly was: a fierce determination. He devoured knowledge not for personal gain, but to help his patients.

The news headlines were filled with statistics of the death tolls around the world. The numbers were slowly creeping up and sadly, many of those numbers included healthcare workers. Our anxieties and fears around the virus soon turned into anger and frustration.

When Mary Agyapong, a 28-year-old nurse, died of Covid-19 shortly after delivering her baby, I was distraught. She worked and died at the same hospital that I was planning to deliver you, Radhika. She lived down the road from us. I later learned that black pregnant women are five times more likely to die during childbirth in this country, and that black and ethnic minority healthcare workers were more likely to contract and then die from Covid-19.

I started to reflect on the reasons for these disparities, pondering why issues such as structural racism weren't being acknowledged, let alone addressed. I decided to take my one-woman protest to Downing Street – a decision that turned my quiet and calm life definitively in the opposite direction.

Your grandparents were deeply uncomfortable with the fact that I was taking a stand. They felt they had an obligation to Britain; after all, it was this very country which allowed them to build their lives and, in my father's case, escape extreme poverty. I faced uncomfortable conversations with family members, trying to reason with them and explain my decisions. At the heart of my anger and frustration was the dreadful realisation that it could have been me. I could have been lying in an intensive care unit bed with you in my womb,

Radhika. I soon realised that everyone chose to live blissfully ignorant to the realities of the circumstances. After all, it was the easiest option.

On a Sunday morning in April, I waddled down Whitehall, carrying my sign, and planted myself in front of the Downing Street gates. My knees tired, but every time I thought about calling it a day, you would remind me to keep going with a gentle kick. In my XXL scrub top, it was hard to tell that I was heavily pregnant as I held a silent vigil outside to honour the memory of Nurse Mary.

On the rare occasion we had a day to ourselves, your father and I would receive communications from some managers who worked at our hospitals, unhappy with what we were doing. While it felt that the public were supporting healthcare workers, there was certainly a movement within the NHS to suppress us.

None of this stopped us from speaking the truth and, eventually, we took a stand against the British government. Your grandparents were terrified for our safety; they were worried about our future and how our actions would eventually impact you, Radhika. But we had no other option because we couldn't allow the suffering that we had witnessed to continue.

To this day, I feel a sense of survivor's guilt knowing that I made it and Mary didn't. I carry her memory everywhere I go.

From the moment I held you, Radhika, all my fears disappeared. From that day, nothing fazed me.

The future, once a looming storm cloud, stretched into a horizon painted with the colours of possibility.

* * *

Anoushka, you were welcomed into the post-pandemic world in February 2024. My birth experience with you was a whole world away from Radhika's birth. I had your father by my side the whole time and your nanny came to the hospital a few hours after you were born to feed me her soft, buttery parathas. I wasn't fearful for our safety and I was so very grateful that we all survived the pandemic to be present for your arrival into this world. You, Anoushka, born under the watchful eye of a pandemic, were a symbol of hope, a testament to our resilience and the sweet reward for all we'd overcome.

I remember kissing your cheeks for the first time and holding your father's hand, trying to make the moment last forever. We all commented on your chubby cheeks and soon came to the realisation that despite trying to open your eyes, your cheeks were hindering your eyelids from opening up!

We smiled, we hugged each other, we laughed, devoid of any fear or uncertainty. I didn't take a single second for granted. You made me believe in miracles again, and you reminded me that love always finds a way to heal.

* * *

Shivika, you arrived in December 2024, a time when our lives had found a new rhythm. It was not without chaos, but there was a deeper sense of feeling settled. You were born into a family already overflowing with love, and your sisters could hardly contain their excitement.

Radhika was the first to hold you, beaming with pride as if she had waited her whole life for that moment. Anoushka whispered gently into your ear, introducing herself with all the seriousness and tenderness of a big sister ready to share her world.

Your birth was calm and beautiful, the kind of calm that only comes after a storm has passed. I remember lying in that hospital bed, your tiny body curled on my chest, and feeling the weight of the past few years lift quietly from my shoulders.

You, Shivika, are the quiet light that slipped into our family like poetry. Unexpected in your softness but profound in your presence. You were born into a world that is still healing, still learning, and still hurting in places, but your arrival reminded me that love renews itself again and again.

You completed us. Not because something was missing before, but because your presence made our family feel fuller, like a symphony that comes alive when all the instruments are finally playing in harmony.

Each of you have healed me in your own way. In your laughter, your tears, your questions and your courage, you have helped me rediscover parts of myself I didn't know were lost. You deserve nothing less than the best of me.

This book is my promise to you, and it is my gift - the story of our journey, with all its trials and triumphs, to inspire your own path in the future.

With love,
Mummy

Chapter 1

EARLY DAYS OF COVID

Confusion and Information Desert

Nishant and I met in a small town in the Czech Republic, far from the familiar comfort of home, as we navigated the strange and unfamiliar world of being international students. The town was quiet, almost serene, and we found solace in the simple joys of life – sport, laughter and each other's company. There were few of us from abroad, and we quickly bonded over our shared experiences. I remember the first time we met, at a squash centre, laughing about how our parents had 'forced' us into medicine, a story familiar to many South Asian children of our generation. It was a light-hearted moment, but one that marked the start of something deeper.

As the cold, snowy days set in, we found warmth in cooking together, experimenting with new recipes as if to bring a little flavour of home into our small, quiet town. In the spring, we'd take long walks along the river, surrounded by the peace and stillness of our surroundings, finding in each other a sense of calm and understanding amid the chaos of our demanding medical studies. Nishant, four years ahead of me in medical school, was often busy preparing for exams and settling into his own journey. By the time he graduated, I still had years left to study while he moved back to the UK to begin his work as a junior doctor.

The distance between us was hard to bear. Social media wasn't as accessible back then, and there were times when we wouldn't speak for days. The silence between us was difficult, but we both carried on with our lives, knowing there was an end goal in sight. While the distance was tough, we had a clear purpose – my focus was on finishing my degree and then finally reuniting with him in the UK. He was starting his career, building his life in the UK, while I was still buried in textbooks. We both faced our own challenges, but there was an unspoken understanding between us – each of us finding our own path, but always supporting the other, no matter how far apart we were.

After four long years, we were finally reunited in the UK. I had started my own journey as a junior doctor, and Nishant had begun his training to become a GP. It was during my first two years as a junior doctor that we decided to start our family.

The early months of my first pregnancy were debilitating. My pregnancy was already far rougher than I had anticipated. My husband, Nishant, was very much au fait with patients like me and he devoted a lot of his time to drip-feeding me juices and smoothies; he was desperate to give me all the nutrition I needed. The vomiting was excruciating, to the extent that I would often have to pull over to the nearest service station on my way to work. My stops at these service stations would often mean that I would be running late for work; an additional stress which only made my nausea worse.

Rhythmical punches and kicks would wake me through

the night, a constant reminder that I was now host to a baby for whom I was totally responsible. Every time there was a jolt of momentary discomfort, I felt as if my baby was checking in to tell me she was okay.

Every morning, in my head, I would re-enact motivational YouTube videos that I would watch at night to help me fall asleep. I would tell myself everything and anything that would help me put one foot in front of the other to make it through the doors of the hospital. Making it to work while feeling sick to my stomach wasn't the most impressive thing I'd achieve on my sickest days; it was my impression of Oprah. I'd go from slurring my words, to raising my voice to a warm and resonant alto in seconds.

I consumed lemon sherbets in excessive amounts as a desperate measure to ease my sickness. My car was littered with sherbet wrappers, and I was constantly embarrassed at my new found addiction. I would find sherbet wrappers everywhere: in my scrub pockets, at my doctor's desk, and sometimes I would even find them underneath my bra strap.

As a doctor, I was reluctant to ever take time off work. I was constantly worried about how my absence would affect my team. We were already short on doctors and if I took time off, I would be adding more stress to the already existing workload my colleagues were faced with. I didn't give myself the grace to think about how I was feeling and what I needed.

I was reluctant to allow pregnancy to make me appear weaker. It wasn't until one of my consultants was adamant about sending me home during one of my ward rounds that I realised I had to listen to my body and rest.

So, I convalesced at home as my bump began to grow. I had plenty of time to mull over my future. I had visions of our first visit with my husband to the sonographer to find out whether we'd be having a boy or a girl. I had visions of my own mother being a birthing partner and being able to share in the joy of seeing her first grandchild. I was entertaining thoughts of a baby shower. I was in a state of constant pre-embarrassment, knowing that my goofy husband would joke around during antenatal classes.

As I waited for my nausea to improve while just about hydrating on an unpalatable cocktail of ginger juice and anti-sickness pills, I imagined returning to work with a visibly bigger bump. I mused on the absurdity of my profession in this new, cumbersome form, imagining myself a slow-motion superhero, incapable of the swift reflexes once demanded of a doctor. I was worried that I would be far too exhausted to function as a doctor.

Towards the end of January my sickness subsided and I returned to work. Cabin fever had overtaken nausea as my primary concern, and I was desperate to help my patients and see my brilliant colleagues once again. I was blissfully ignorant to the fact that I would soon be in the eye of a storm.

As I continued working into February, my husband would return from his own night shifts and tell me stories of unusual cases in Accident & Emergency (A&E). He didn't seem too concerned when recounting these cases to me. He was told to be extra cautious when seeing these patients and would follow the personal protective gear guidelines like we normally do in the NHS. Everything seemed as if it was under control; there was no reason to feel otherwise. After all, our nation takes great pride in having one of the best healthcare systems in the world.

At that time, we were following the news on how the

coronavirus had hit China hard, but it still felt like another world away. I was trying to arrange a gazebo and catering for my baby shower, and I knew that nothing could ever happen to me. Not in this country, not on these shores.

In March, as my sickness had eased, I started to see a steady stream of patients with presumed coronavirus. I was five months pregnant and working 12-hour shifts in a hyper-anxious state, with variable access to masks. There was a general state of denial throughout the hospital, but as the tsunami crossed Asia and hit Italy, then Spain, then France, it seemed inevitable that we would be impacted. Worryingly, there was no data and little guidance regarding pregnant women at that time.

* * *

In March 2020, there were 3912 deaths involving the coronavirus in the UK. This was a number that I wasn't able to visualise, as seeing just one death on any of my shifts would take a huge emotional toll. The prospect of witnessing such a cataclysmic loss multiplied by thousands was a nightmare beyond comprehension.

These were real human lives that were lost. This wasn't just about the numbers; this was about the thousands of people whose lives changed overnight after losing a loved one. This number is an underestimate and the real number could have been much higher as the government decided to cease community testing very early on in the pandemic.

Nishant had the foresight and knowledge to predict this outcome in March 2020 as he kept alluding to the possibility that we were heading towards a disaster situation. During his shifts in A&E, he noticed how policies on infection control kept changing. In February 2020, he was told to wear a full hazmat suit to see patients with presumed coronavirus. Nishant would come home telling me stories about how the hazmat suits were a great ice-breaker for his younger patients in A&E. Overnight, his stories went from funny anecdotes about hazmat suits, to frightening accounts of having to admit his own colleagues into the intensive care unit as they were becoming unwell.

NHS policy has always been very strict on infection control. Doctors and nurses are often penalised for wearing anything below the elbow, including nail varnish. Many of us would tie our watches around our lanyards with the knowledge that an infection control nurse could walk past us any time and discipline us. Although many of us would find this frustrating, it was necessary to avoid cross-contamination between doctors and patients.

If we were functioning in a system which played such close attention to detail when it came to infection control and patient safety, how and why did we get things so catastrophically wrong?

Working in highly infectious areas and caring for symptomatic patients made us the main vectors of transmission. It very rapidly became obvious in the coronavirus pandemic that the priority should have been to protect healthcare workers. We soon started to realise that the supply of protective gear was a global problem, and global supply chains of personal protective equipment (PPE) were drying up quickly. Countries were competing for the supply of goods in a way that we hadn't really seen before.

As the coronavirus cast its insidious net across the globe, a frantic scramble for PPE ensued. Supply chains, once robust and reliable, snapped under the immense pressure, leaving nations and healthcare systems desperately rationing precious resources. Rationing became the grim new norm, forcing medical professionals into a macabre form of triage, deciding who would wear what scant protection. In this bleak landscape, doctors and nurses transformed into ghostly figures, shrouded in makeshift armour – bin bags serving as flimsy shields against an invisible enemy. The desperation deepened as even the most basic of safeguards became luxuries, with healthcare workers resorting to repurposing children's science goggles for protection.

According to research by the Royal Society of Medicine, three billion pieces of PPE were used by the NHS in just the first six months of the crisis.[1] However, the Department for Health and Social Care accounts for 2020/21 reveal that £673m worth of PPE bought during the pandemic was unusable,[2] while £750m of equipment was not used before its expiry date.

Unfortunately, the supply of personal protective gear wasn't the only issue crippling the ability of the NHS to protect the British public; there weren't enough tests to go around. One major roadblock the NHS was facing at the time was the lack of testing. It seems very obvious now, but any member of the public who showed any symptoms of the virus should have been tested for Covid-19. This way, it would have been very clear and easy to identify if anybody walking through the doors of the hospital was positive or not.

Still, in the early stages of the outbreak in February 2020, Britain appeared to be coping well with identifying infected patients and doing contact tracing. When the first two cases were identified in the northern city of York at the end of January, health officials put them into isolation and traced their contacts. The same was done for a man from Brighton, who had travelled to Singapore and then France before returning home and infecting four people.

It didn't become clear until later, when confirmed cases began to increase exponentially in early March, that Britain's failure to move fast on obtaining testing kits back in February would have such a big impact.

The UK government made a string of controversial decisions in mid-March. The first came on 12 March, the day after the World Health Organization (WHO) declared Covid-19 a pandemic, when public health officials announced that the UK would cease tracing and testing the contacts of coronavirus patients.

The decision to stop community testing was against WHO advice, which was that you need to 'test, test, test'.

11 March: The health secretary Matt Hancock had declared that the government was 'rolling out a big expansion of testing' but there were no specific numbers or timelines given.

12 March: Boris Johnson announced that healthcare workers, which included GPs, would no longer test people for the virus in their homes, but would continue to test people already in hospitals.

16 March: The World Health Organization Director General Tedros Adhanom Ghebreyesus had one message to countries across the world: 'Test, test, test.' He warned that countries could not 'fight a fire blindfolded'.

I fully appreciate the gravity of the situation and how in reality, no country could have been fully prepared for the pandemic. As with any health crisis, any new rules or regulations which are set in place must be backed up with reasonable evidence. Unfortunately, Public Health England (PHE) did not publish any evidence as to why community testing was stopped during the pandemic in March 2020.

To summarise, this is what was happening mid-March 2020:

- The UK was expecting a tsunami of cases to come into NHS hospitals, yet there was not enough equipment to deal with those who would be critically unwell.
- Community testing had stopped, so nobody knew who was walking through the doors of A&E.
- Nishant, and quite possibly many other doctors across the country, predicted that we would witness a great deal of suffering if our government ministers didn't follow scientific advice and evidence. All our concerns were travelling into a void – nobody would listen.
- There were no official guidelines regarding the safety of pregnant women in a clinical setting and in the community.

No country was prepared for the pandemic. The role of the government was to minimise the risk and scale of suffering for the British public. This was all possible, if only it had acted on the shocking data and statistics it had been sitting on for years.

* * *

In 2016, the government carried out a simulation, Exercise Cygnus. It was done with a view to predict how Britain would respond to a flu pandemic. It recruited 950 ministers, officials and civil servants to role-play how the machinery of government would cope with the pressures of a major outbreak of a novel disease. The report on Exercise Cygnus[3] warned that the UK was not prepared for a pandemic.

During this exercise, officials were told to put themselves in the shoes of a minister dealing with the seventh week of a pandemic. This would be a point where there would be a peak in demand for social and hospital care. This whole exercise was not only to test how emergencies would be dealt with under strain, but to also acclimatise ministers and officials to dealing with high-pressure situations and managing their decision-making process.

The report stated that 'the UK's preparedness and response, in terms of its plans, policies and capability, is currently not sufficient to cope with the extreme demands of a severe pandemic that will have a nationwide impact across all sectors'.

One problem identified during this exercise was that while each government body in the exercise had reasonable plans, enabling a decentralised response, nobody in the centre had oversight over everyone else.

The impact of this lack of preparedness was significant. The report was produced in July 2017 and sent out to all major government departments and NHS England. The results of Exercise Cygnus were leaked to *The Guardian* newspaper in May 2020. A complete version was later released in October 2020 by the Department of Health and Social Care[4] after public pressure.

Surprisingly, Exercise Cygnus was not the only simulation carried out to test the capacity of the NHS for a pandemic. This was just one of ten unpublicised pandemic exercises carried out in the five years before Covid-19, all of which were kept secret until pressure from doctors and the public forced the Department of Health and Social Care to reveal their findings.

The other exercises carried out included simulations to prepare for Ebola, influenza, Lassa fever, bird flu, and there was also one exercise that dealt with a radiation incident nicknamed Exercise Cerberus.

Just four years before the pandemic hit us, the government had all the data and information it needed to ensure the country wouldn't be heading towards a disaster. Specifically, Exercise Cygnus reported a serious shortage of ventilators and PPE. This lack of transparency directly impacted the mortality rate and, worst of all, it was clear from these exercises that the lack of PPE was a pinch point in the country's preparation for the pandemic.

The UK, a leading country in many scientific fields, couldn't get the basics of pandemic preparation right. I could have never imagined it. We all expected hiccups at the start as the government was trying to plan for the pandemic. Yet, the subsequent paralysis, a stagnant pool of inaction amid a sea of data, has cast an enduring shadow over the very fabric of British politics.

* * *

I was sitting in my living room on a Sunday morning, enjoying a warm coffee and trying to make the most of my free weekend. It was a refreshing change from drinking cold, instant coffee from a plastic cup in my doctor's office. My hospital coffees were always made just warm enough to trick myself into believing that I was enjoying a hot drink, but also easy to gulp within two sips in case of any emergency. The unique flavour of my hospital coffees was the after-taste of a wooden stirrer which, sadly, I got used to after working in the NHS for a couple of years.

I was gently caressing my belly, eagerly trying to provoke my baby into a combative kick or punch. In between midwife appointments and hospital shifts, it didn't feel as if there was much time to absorb the tender moments of my pregnancy. I had imagined this moment for many years. I was finally settled: married, a steady job, pregnant with my first child. Stability didn't come easy, and it was earned through a series of acutely painful rites of passage.

'Kings Cross Station. Meeting with Carole Cadwalladr. ETA 1pm.'

Nishant's text jolted me out of my belly-rubbing bubble. It seemed unusual that he had scheduled an impromptu meeting with an investigative journalist. Our Sundays were a sacred ritual, a leisurely ballet of coffee and companionship. He loved to lie in on a Sunday morning. In fact, it was an unwritten rule in our house: wake up at leisure and enjoy the signature coffee at our local cafe. Nishant's order was always a large Americano and I'd mix my orders up between either a cappuccino or flat white. I still can't tell the difference between both, probably because I always have coffee with my sugar rather than the other way around.

Immediately, I went into a rabbit hole of googling Carole. I found tweets and articles predicting the impact of the virus hitting the UK and the growing statistics of the death toll across the world. At this point, there were 35 deaths in the UK and 1140 confirmed cases. Countries were closing their borders and mass gatherings were showing a clear spike in cases. Our worst fears were about to become a reality: the UK was about to shut down, and despite attempting to take such extreme measures at the eleventh hour, it was too little too late.

My eyes were fixated on my phone screen and within moments, I transported myself into an apocalyptic scenario where the NHS had run out of hospital beds and epidural kits due to the pandemic. Before I knew it, I was planning a home birth where I was left alone with no family around to support me. This was a fear which always lingered in my mind but I was never brave enough to entertain it. Although this was my worst-case scenario, it was becoming my most likely scenario and it terrified me.

As I put my feet back up on the sofa and grounded myself back into my pregnancy bubble, my husband was sitting in one of the most important meetings of his life. A meeting that would overturn our perfectly planned months ahead of us.

Nishant had seemed distant in the weeks leading up to his meeting with Carole. Initially, it upset me that he seemed less interested in engaging in our husband-wife activities. Our evening marathons of watching *The Thick of It* turned into watching the news, and our evening catch-ups were replaced with discussions about Nishant's Covid-19 patients in A&E. The long commute to work was taking a toll on my pregnant body and Nishant's cognitive load would reach its limit by the end of the day.

I felt that his demeanour was justified by our circumstances; we were both trying to survive long shifts in the hospital and the weight of uncertainty of the virus was a big burden to carry. Our minds were miles apart; I was daydreaming of welcoming our baby girl into this world, while Nishant spent every second of his day disaster planning.

As I resumed massaging my belly and blissfully ignoring everything that I had just read, I turned on the TV to distract myself further. My distraction strategy didn't quite work out because the TV opened up on Sky News. Tedros Adhanom Ghebreyesus, Director General of the World Health Organization, was speaking at a press conference. At the bottom of the screen, on the scrolling ticker, I read: 'Coronavirus: NHS staff urge PM to provide more protective equipment as two consultants receive critical care.'[5]

The news report explored the distress that doctors were experiencing due to the lack of access to PPE within NHS trusts. What had shocked me the most was learning that doctors who were working in intensive care units were using masks that had expired back in 2015.

Doctors weren't receiving adequate PPE and it was clear that they were getting very sick. There was a glaringly obvious correlation which couldn't be missed; doctors were getting sick because they didn't have the correct protective gear. At this point (16 March 2020), there were reports of two consultants who were on ventilators in intensive care after contracting the virus. Reading this headline took me back to the time when I was desperately pleading for work adjustments for my pregnancy. What if, like me, other doctors were asking for help, only to end up in a system flooded with requests and emails?

The NHS at the time had about 8000 ventilators available, but scientific modelling, based on evidence from China, had suggested that up to 30,000 ventilators would be needed within a matter of weeks. On 16 March, the same day Nishant had gone to speak to Carole Cadwalladr, it was announced on the news that medical device specialists were asked to launch a wartime-style effort to bridge the gap in ventilators.

After meeting Carole, Nishant came straight home and walked through the door at around midday. The sun was shining, it was Sunday, and all I really wanted to do was go for a walk in our local park and stop by our favourite coffee place. Before I could even suggest this to Nishant, he threw himself on the sofa, opened his laptop and started typing away.

I offered Nishant lunch and suggested we could sit in the garden and talk about what had happened that morning with Carole. He agreed to the suggestion, and when I did serve lunch, he went back to the sofa and continued on his laptop. We exchanged a few words that morning and although I knew that his meeting with Carole was not to be taken lightly, I tried to ignore it. I was too scared to entertain any thoughts of the pandemic overturning our lives.

Nishant and I were on completely different wavelengths. I wanted to eat lunch in the garden, sip on a flat white and update my Instagram profile about my pregnancy. Nishant, on the other hand, was on a mission to send a wake-up call to the world that the virus would kill us all if we didn't take things seriously.

'Nishant, I think you're taking this too far and might be overreacting.' I tried to calmly explain to Nishant that putting his neck on the line wouldn't save the country. At least that's what I thought at the time. The weight of this immense responsibility threatened to eclipse our domestic haven, casting a long shadow over our newborn and our fragile family unit.

'Meenal, people will die. Our parents might die. You might die and we might never see our baby,' Nishant explained in frustration.

Even when Nishant mentioned the possible catastrophe that could hit our families, I still didn't feel a sense of urgency being injected in me. Perhaps in some way, I took my life for granted. I was always taken care of when I was unwell; I never had to worry about the NHS running out of medicines or machines to take care of me because the resources had always been readily available.

'Meenal, a lot of people will find out that you're pregnant tonight. Family in the UK, possibly family in India and, well, anybody who reads Carole's article in *The Guardian*,' Nishant warned me.

'Yes, but our family will get upset if I don't call them up myself and tell them.' I was worried about how our family would react.

It wasn't acceptable in our South Asian families for any pregnancy to be announced in such a casual manner. It had to be done with rituals and centuries-old traditions in place. It definitely wasn't acceptable to bear the good news through a news article, widely available to the public. Nishant had made a very conscious decision to pour his energy only into what had mattered at the time. He refused to entertain any conversation around family politics and rightly so. He was only concerned about sending out a powerful message to the British public: we had a great deal of suffering coming our way over the next few months if our politicians continued to respond with such apathy and carelessness.

This was my first pregnancy. I always dreamed of announcing the news with all our family members gathered around our dinner table, opening customised gifts and a cake big enough to feed our whole neighbourhood. I wanted an announcement that would have looked great on Instagram, not a news headline discussing the potential deaths of thousands of people within the next few weeks.

Reluctantly, Nishant agreed to go for a walk with me. We went down our local high street and his pace was a lot faster than usual. It seemed to me that he just wanted to get this walk done and out of the way so he could go back to his laptop at home. As we were walking, I tried to keep up with him and find ways to slow him down to my penguin waddle-like pace. I held his hand but it would just slip away as he carried on walking. In an attempt to lighten up the mood, I nervously tried to joke around. I had very little understanding of what Nishant was trying to achieve but I knew I had to support him. In all the years I've known Nishant, I've watched him face some challenging situations, but this felt different. His eyes were heavy with worry and there was an urgency in his step. For the first time in our marriage, I felt helpless. I was desperate to support him, but didn't know how to. Over time, this cloud of guilt would follow and consume me. There was nobody I could speak to because we were in such a unique position; who else could relate to having a whistleblower husband?

As we were walking, I noticed that our local TK Maxx was open and it had an offer on baby clothes. Although Nishant was in a perpetual state of exhaustion and worry, there was one thing that always brought a smile to his face: picturing the arrival of our baby girl and adorning her in the prettiest floral and colourful dresses.

This seemed like a good escape from wherever Nishant's mind was wandering. As we got to the baby aisle, Nishant's eyes started to brighten up and he seemed more engaged in talking about something other than the virus. For a moment, I felt a sense of normality. This was it. This was what I wanted this whole time – to unapologetically enjoy these precious moments before the arrival of our baby girl.

It almost felt too good to be true. So I picked up a boy's outfit and asked Nishant what he thought of it. When he replied, 'I'm pretty sure that's for boys', I laughed with relief that Nishant was present in the moment with me.

We continued down the aisle and we argued over the colour of our baby girl's first onesie. I had no specific preference, but I wanted to make this moment fun and enjoyable because I knew this wouldn't last forever. Unfortunately, it only lasted a few moments and after exchanging a few smiles and jokes, Nishant received a phone call from *The Guardian* editors. They wanted to take headshots of Nishant straight away as they were planning to publish the article that same evening.

Nishant dropped everything at the store and held my hand to walk straight back home. I reminded myself that this would all be over soon and within a few days, maybe we could come back to this same store and carry on where we left off. As we made our way home, I stopped Nishant and squeezed his hand.

'Please tell me exactly what is going on. You're taking this too far. It's just a virus; you can't fix everything.'

'You don't get it, Meenal. Nobody gets it.'

He was right. Nobody understood the severity of the situation because a lot of information was hidden from the public at the time. Nishant let go of my hand in frustration and walked straight home. I sat on the bench and wondered when all of this would be over. We were on the brink of lockdown and so many unknowns. It was terrifying. At that moment, I decided that I wouldn't allow this fear to consume me. I knew Nishant needed my full support and, as his wife, I just had to show up. All of my questions could have been answered later.

* * *

'"Everyone is scared to speak up": A&E doctor asks for Covid-19 tests.' This was the news headline that was released by *The Guardian* that evening on 16 March; a stark, unforgiving indictment. It was around 6pm and Nishant had a shift starting in A&E at 9pm that night. We were in London, as we had been to visit Nishant's parents for the weekend, and on the Sunday evening we faced a one-hour drive to get home.

As soon as the article came out, a stream of notifications started to flood my phone. I had over 20 messages from close friends and family popping up on my phone with a range of reactions:

'Is this your husband, Meenal? He's so brave.'

'Congratulations on the pregnancy. It would have been nice to have received a phone call at least.'

'Nishant is overreacting; we'll be fine!'

'You have to be really careful, Meenal. Nishant might lose his job; he can't speak up like this.'

'I had no idea you were pregnant. Take care of yourself and be safe.'

This last message was a gentle reminder that despite all the chaos and doom around us, I was allowed to think about myself and it was okay if at any point I decided to put myself and my baby first.

Nishant clearly wasn't in the right headspace to drive. Of course, that was a very natural reaction for someone in his position. Despite the fears and worries crowding in on him in that moment, he still had clarity in his thought process. This is something I always admire about Nishant; nothing fazes him when it comes to making life-changing decisions.

During our drive, Nishant was glued to his phone. He was receiving messages from colleagues concerned about potential fallout from the article. Although his news article made no comments on his specific hospital or trust and was aimed mainly at the structural issues affecting the NHS, we believed that he could be in trouble. Nishant had thoroughly researched past whistleblower cases within the NHS and other major global organizations, and a clear pattern emerged – the consequences for those who spoke out were often severe, with outcomes that could be punitive and unjust.

That night, as we were driving down the motorway, I realised that this was a testing time for us as a couple. As he held my hand, a silent promise passed between us. Beneath the calm exterior, I knew his mind was a tempest, torn between duty and the looming spectre of upheaval. His bravery was a beacon, but the shadow of potential chaos stretched long and dark. Nishant knew that, although he had acted on principle and felt it was necessary to speak up. His voice, a gentle counterpoint to the rushing wind, carried a quiet strength. He acknowledged the looming shadow of potential upheaval, a stark realisation that could shatter our world.

As his wife, I felt I had a duty not just to support him, but also to understand why this was so important to him. Both of us had a baby coming along the way and we had an exciting few months ahead of us. Why did he want to throw all of that away and put his neck on the line?

It seemed at that point, there was no winning for us; we were up against a British Institution consisting of highly experienced PR teams and politicians who knew very well how to manipulate facts and figures to favour their own narrative.

That evening, I felt we had made a huge mistake. I knew it was important and I was acutely aware of the implications of not speaking up, but what if Nishant lost his job? What if we'd thrown our future away in the search for accountability and justice? We had worked so incredibly hard to become doctors; our families sacrificed everything they had to financially support us. This one misstep could have thrown all of that away.

I was clearly terrified of facing the consequences, but Nishant had calculated everything he possibly could. Every potential outcome was a landmine waiting to explode. He knew that as he walked into work, there was a chance that he might be taken into a room with his senior colleagues for a chat. He was also prepared to get sent home straight away. Yet, in the face of this looming catastrophe, an eerie calm washed over him.

The one-hour drive felt like an eternity. Nishant squeezed my hand as he left the car and said, 'I'll see you in the morning. Make sure you get some rest. We've had a long day.'

Both of us knew that neither of us would get any rest that night.

Chapter 2

THE ROOTS OF MY ACTIVISM

My mother was born and raised in New Delhi. As the eldest of three, she was born under the watchful gaze of a society steeped in tradition. She had two younger brothers and was constantly reminded of the path expected of her – a life woven from household chores and the quiet hum of domesticity. Yet, within her, a tiny flame flickered, a spark of something more, something different.

My maternal grandparents lived through the tail end of the British Raj and witnessed the devastating Partition of India. My grandmother has very few memories of her time during the Partition but she remembers living in makeshift tents with her four other siblings at the border between India and Pakistan. The land, the very foundation of their family home, painstakingly built by her great grandfather, was swallowed whole by the Partition. Each time she speaks of those days, a tremor runs through her voice, a reminder of the suffering that ripped through families and communities. Theirs was just one story in a million, a testament to the enduring scars left by the British Raj.

My grandmother was only 17 years old when she got married to my grandfather and, at that time, young girls were groomed from a very young age to be prepared for marriage. She barely remembers going to school, but has very clear memories of learning how to cook and clean in preparation of raising her own family. Her youthful dreams, if they ever existed, were carefully tucked away, replaced by the realities of enacting her wifely duties.

My grandfather went through a very similar experience. Millions of families were displaced during this period and my grandfather lost his father at a very young age. During the displacement of Hindus and Muslims, many settled in Delhi and that's where my grandparents were married and raised their family. My grandfather became an engineer, building not just structures, but a future for his family. Though their lives were shaped by the upheaval of the Partition, a shared resilience bloomed within them. They were a testament to the enduring spirit, a love story born from the ashes of displacement. Their Delhi home, though a far cry from their roots, became a sanctuary.

I have little information on the generations before my grandparents. But with my grandparents as the starting point, a picture emerges – a world where education for girls was a flickering candle flame, easily snuffed out. Here, family values were a tightly woven net, designed to keep women in their designated place. My mother, however, dared to step out of the preordained circle, and was the first woman in our family to do so. While her younger cousins married at the tender age of 17, my mother craved a different path – a career in teaching geography. She clung to her dream of a later marriage, a life built on her own terms. Her story became a beacon, a testament to the courage it takes to break free from the shackles of expectation, to forge a path where none existed before. It was a legacy she would one day pass on.

Her determination and willingness to break this cycle allowed me to become a doctor. My upbringing wasn't burdened by the weight of tradition. Instead, it bloomed with independence and the unshakeable belief that I could achieve anything. Now, as I raise my daughters, I feel the weight on my own shoulders is a little bit lighter. Their world is a canvas waiting to be painted, and I can guide them with the knowledge that they are free to choose their own paths. My mother's courage and her legacy which she has passed down will empower my daughters to break free from any limitations.

The weight of history still rests on us. My mother, though limited by the choices of the past, still dared to forge a new path.

My father grew up in a less privileged family. He was raised in the slums of New Delhi. He experienced the sting of hunger and the hollowness of an empty stomach. School books were a luxury and electricity a distant dream. Yet, under the harsh glare of streetlights, my father devoured knowledge and would sit on the side roads and read books that he had found in the neighbourhood's rubbish pile. He prioritised his family, ensuring they had food even if his own meals were scraps from roadside vendors. This wasn't life, it was a relentless cycle, but my father always dreamed of breaking free.

My father was one of eight siblings, but he was different from them all. His brilliance caught the eye of his headmaster, who offered him a lifeline – a scholarship that would propel him beyond the dusty alleys. Every day began at 3am, and before the sun peeked over the horizon, my father would collect vegetables, set up the family stall, and then sprint to school with his textbooks clutched under his arm.

Between balancing the dire financial situation of his family and his schoolwork, my father became a chartered accountant. Financial freedom, once a distant dream, finally bought him the power to shield his family from hardship. He'd devour newspapers, London and Europe splashed across the pages, igniting a yearning to step foot on those distant lands. Pictures of Wembley Stadium filled him with awe – a monument to a world he yearned to experience. 'Maybe my grandchildren,' he'd joke with friends, 'will have the luxury of seeing it in person.'

His twenties were a blur of relentless hustle. He built a life for his family in Gibraltar, a stark contrast to the straw hut of his childhood. I remember the day he held the key to his first property. I was only 11 years old, and tears welled in his eyes as the realisation of his hard work and suffering washed over him. Now, he could provide for his family, build a home that wasn't woven from straw. He could finally breathe; he'd finally made it.

My father's story is a testament to the enduring human spirit. My proudest moment was taking him to Wembley after I received the Lionhearts award for my work during the pandemic. This wasn't just a dream come true for him; it was the culmination of a life dedicated to breaking cycles, and a powerful reminder that the ripples of our efforts can touch generations to come.

* * *

I was never encouraged to speak my heart out as a child.

Unlike my friends, whose homes echoed with open dialogues about dreams and anxieties, mine felt like a fortress with walls built of unspoken expectations. I craved that same freedom, that safe harbour where emotions could flow freely. This disparity gnawed at me. My friends, with their open hearts and unfiltered voices, seemed to navigate life with a confidence I craved. They argued with their parents (good-naturedly, of course) about curfews and career choices. I, on the other hand, bottled everything up and accepted the role of being a silent observer. The stifling silence within me became a silent vow, a promise to one day find my voice, even if it meant learning to speak in the language of courage.

As a teenager, I wanted to question so many things but I was always told to stop wasting my time and just focus on my school and exams and get good grades. I remember my mother once telling me that being so curious wouldn't get me anywhere; it would only bring me more trouble. And of course, as the daughter of the family, I couldn't be the troublemaker. Isolated in this sea of unquestioning acceptance, I lacked the tools to navigate the currents of critical thought. Information washed over me, each piece accepted as truth without a ripple of doubt. My voice, a tiny spark of rebellion, remained trapped within, yearning to break free. But the fear of causing a commotion, of being labelled a 'troublemaker', kept it firmly muted. The cost of conformity, though silent, was a heavy one.

That was the total opposite of what I needed in March 2020. If I wanted to save lives, I had to critically analyse where things were going wrong. Throughout my period of campaigning and protesting, my mother's anxiety wasn't about the repercussions of my actions; it was the potential judgement swirling around my own, then-unknown, pregnancy. I needed her to see the bigger picture, to understand that sometimes, doing the right thing comes at a social cost.

There is a saying in Hindi, '*Log kya kehenge*', which directly translates to 'What will people say?' It was the unwelcome guest at every decision table. Did I dare wear a skirt that danced a few inches above the knee? *Log kya kehenge?* The yearning to travel and explore the world before heading to university was met with the same weary refrain. *Log kya kehenge?*

This insidious phrase, a weapon of mass conformity, had become the executioner of countless dreams. It silenced ambitions, strangled aspirations. This phrase, a weapon wielded by well-meaning but fearful hearts, became a graveyard for aspirations. It silenced the whispers of possibility, the yearnings for experiences beyond the confines of our community. It was a chorus of voices, dictating the script of our lives. Every time I was making life-changing decisions, I would hear the whispers of '*log kya kehenge*', but I also heard the courageous roar of my own heart.

Confidence, a flower that once bloomed readily, wilted under the harsh glare of cultural expectations. The 'what will people say?' became a constant internal battle cry, chipping away at me.

Perhaps, if the burden of reputation hadn't been so heavy, I could have faced the world with a lighter step and with a clearer mind. But even with the lingering anxieties, the flame of hope flickered on. This wasn't just about protecting my family's reputation; it was about creating a new legacy, one built on love, acceptance, and the freedom to write our own stories. It was a battle I was determined to fight, not just for myself, but for the generations to come. I know that if I asked myself what society thought about my actions during the time I decided to protest, I would have let more deaths and suffering slip in front of my eyes.

I remember my father desperately trying to talk me out of the protest: 'Meenal, these politicians are much more powerful than you are. All it takes is one phone call from them and your career is ruined. We've worked too hard for you to throw it all away.'

We were kicked out of our homeland once as a family, and my parents feared history would repeat itself. Was I risking not just my future, but the fragile security we had painstakingly rebuilt?

* * *

Life, I'm realising, is a mosaic. Every decision, big or small, is a tile I placed, slowly building the picture of who I am today. From the school I chose, a stepping stone to knowledge, to the teachers who became guiding lights, each piece has shaped the person I've become. The path that led me here wasn't a straight line, but a labyrinth of choices. Each turn, each decision, led me closer to the person I was meant to be. From the teachers who sparked a fire in my soul, to the school that nurtured my curiosity, every step was a brushstroke on the canvas of my life.

Until I was 18, my world was a bubble. Unburdened by financial woes, my path to becoming a doctor felt pre-ordained, paved with my parents' unwavering support. My parents nurtured the doctor-to-be within me. Then as I applied to medical schools across the UK, the university rejections came crashing down, shattering the illusion. Life, it seemed, had a different script in mind.

I applied to five medical schools in the UK back in 2011 and despite achieving top results in my GCSEs and A-levels, the acceptance letters I craved never arrived. I had received a scholarship from the Government of Gibraltar for my grades, a supposed crown jewel for my academic achievements, but still, this wasn't enough to get me into medical school.

I remember the despair I felt at the time. My emotional toolbox, woefully inadequate, offered no way to navigate this despair. The joy radiating from my friends, planning their dream university courses, felt like a cruel spotlight on my own shattered aspirations. I never failed. I always came home with excellent grades, I was at the top of my class for all my subjects and I dedicated every single day to making sure I got into medical school.

My parents only had one dream – for their daughter to become the first doctor in the family. At the time, I was ready to accept whatever my parents suggested was the next best option. They played with the option of studying a different degree altogether and then looking into the possibility of studying medicine later down the line. The idea of me not going to university at 18 terrified them because it didn't fit in with the path they had planned for me. Their meticulously plotted path – birth, school, university, marriage – had no room for detours. They had no plan B; it was either plan A or nothing at all.

My parents were drowning in their own desperation. There were calls to distant relatives in India and Pakistan, a desperate search for a backdoor route to medicine. My mother took all her jewellery out of her cupboards to see how much she could sell to pay for international fees if I were to study abroad. My father was ready to sell the house he had built with his life's earnings and savings – a testament to the lengths he'd go to fulfil their meticulously crafted dream. I felt obligated to accept their plans, to become the doctor they envisioned, even if it meant selling the very roof over our heads.

One evening, I came back from school and switched on the local news on TV. An advert showed up for an initiative started by the British Government in the UK called 'Volunteer Services Overseas' (VSO). They were recruiting young adults to travel to deprived areas of the world and engage with local communities in Africa and Asia. One year. All expenses covered. Just an application and an interview stood between me and this unexpected adventure. It felt like a lifeline had been thrown at me, and a tiny spark of rebellion ignited within me.

Suddenly, the carefully constructed map of my life, meticulously drawn by my parents, felt stifling. A yearning for something beyond the familiar borders of Gibraltar bloomed within me. This wasn't just about defiance; it was about exploration. A desire to see how others lived, a chance to play a small, but meaningful, role in the lives of the less fortunate. This was a chance to contribute, to write my own story, one adventure at a time.

The application form practically filled itself out. My fingers flew across the keyboard, fuelled by a spark of rebellion I hadn't known existed. Telling my parents? Not a chance. The sting of university rejections was still fresh and I didn't want to burden them with another potential disappointment. Besides, after a lifetime of following their meticulously paved path, this felt like a tiny act of claiming my own agency.

The path of least resistance might have been tempting, but the call of the unknown was far too loud to ignore.

A week crawled by and each day was a tense negotiation between hope and fear. A letter had come through our mailbox and my father got his hands on it first.

'Explain yourself,' he said sternly.

Weren't my parents aiming for the same thing – to help those less fortunate? Maybe a stethoscope wasn't the only tool for healing. But just then, the VSO advert flickered back to life in my mind. Faces, etched with hardship yet alive with hope, swam before me. These weren't problems I could solve, not single-handedly. But maybe, just maybe, I could be a small ripple in the vast ocean of need. After all, wasn't that what they'd always wanted for me too? To be a doctor wasn't just about securing a safe future; it was about service, about easing the burdens of others. I felt this was a chance to make my own mark on the world, a chance to honour their dream while writing a chapter of my own story.

I explained everything to my father and showed him all the work that was previously carried out by VSO on the internet. I had to emphasise that he was the lucky one who escaped the slums of New Delhi. It was a gamble, reminding him of his own past, hoping it would spark empathy and not anger. After a lot of negotiation and late-night conversations with my parents, they hesitantly agreed to let me take a gap year and travel to Mozambique with VSO. For me, it was a doorway flung open to the unknown, a chance to carve my own path, one that started with helping others.

This wasn't just a gap year; it was a baptism by fire. It was a humbling realisation that the world I knew, the one where textbooks held all the answers, was just a sliver of the human experience. It was a seed planted deep within me, a seed that would later bloom into a fierce dedication to social justice. Mozambique wasn't just a place on a map; it was the turning point, the catalyst that propelled me on a lifelong journey of discovery, a journey that began with a single, life-altering step.

I lived with a host family in Chibuto, a small village in the south of Mozambique. It was a world far removed from my parents' overprotective grip. Chibuto was a stark contrast to the life I knew. All I had was a flimsy hope that a local SIM card and a shaky phone signal would bridge the physical and emotional distance between me and my parents. It was a leap of faith, for them and for me, into the unknown.

I travelled with a group of eight other volunteers, all from different walks of life. We were eight souls united by a shared yearning. We were an unlikely orchestra, each member bringing a unique melody to the chorus of our shared purpose. Some, fresh-faced graduates brimming with idealism. Others, veterans of the working world, seeking a respite from the daily grind. Yet, a common thread bound us – a yearning to break free from the familiar and contribute to a world beyond our own. This wasn't just a group of volunteers; it was a microcosm of humanity, united by the desire to make a difference, one hand at a time.

When we first landed in Mozambique, I felt a big rush of humid air hit my skin. Sticky heat clung to my skin like a second shirt, and the cacophony of the airport buzzed with a foreign energy. Every familiar face, every comforting corner of my life, was a world away. Here, in the heart of Mozambique, the enormity of my decision slammed into me. A wave of doubt threatened to drown me – had I been a fool to step outside the sheltered world I knew? I told myself that turning back now wouldn't erase the medical school rejections or rewrite my future. It would simply leave me stranded, adrift in a sea of 'what ifs'. The fear wouldn't vanish entirely, but courage, I realised, wasn't the absence of fear, but the willingness to move forward despite it.

Before I knew it, I was in a white van with all the other volunteers, crammed shoulder-to-shoulder as we jostled along red dirt roads. My visits to Indian villages with family had been glimpses from a car window, sanitised views that offered no preparation for the reality that awaited me here. This wasn't a sightseeing tour; it was a plunge into a new reality, and with every bump and jostle of the van, the enormity of that reality settled in.

When we arrived, a cluster of figures materialised. The village elders were ready to welcome us, their faces etched with the wisdom of a thousand sunrises. Naively, I assumed Portuguese, the official language, would be our bridge. Yet, their greetings were in a language unknown to me.

As introductions began, I was called to greet 'Mama Veronica'. She approached with a smile as warm as the midday sun. Her arms opened wide, and, caught in the moment, I returned the embrace. A torrent of Xitswa flowed from her lips, a language utterly foreign to my ears. In that instant, a wave of isolation washed over me. But Mama Veronica, oblivious to my internal monologue, simply chuckled and patted my hand. Though words failed us, her warmth spoke volumes. With a silent understanding, I offered to carry my luggage, a small gesture in a new language of its own – the language of helping hands and open hearts. The journey had only just begun, and here, on the threshold of a world unknown, a lesson in the universality of human connection was waiting to be learned.

Mama Veronica, her smile a beacon of warmth, ushered me inside her home. The room was a testament to essentials. A single, thin mattress lay sprawled on the dusty floor, remnants of brick construction raining down from the exposed ceiling. A single socket, precariously dangling from the wall, seemed to present a question: 'Do you dare plug anything in?' And then, the final piece of the picture – a large, circular bucket nestled beside the mattress. It was then that the reality of my situation hit me. A bucket. Not a porcelain throne, not a symphony of flushing water, but a bucket. In that moment, the urge to reach for my phone, to dial my dad's number and plead for a one-way ticket back to civilisation, felt overwhelming. This definitely wasn't the glamorous gap year adventure I'd envisioned. But then, Mama Veronica seemed to sense I was uncomfortable, and her smile expressed her willingness to help me through this daunting process.

The room, stripped bare to its earthen essentials, felt like a prison cell. Tears welled up, blurring the scene outside my window. A deflated football, more patches than leather, sailed through the dusty air, propelled by the joyous shrieks of children. Nearby, a group of elders sat huddled around a radio. Their weathered faces, etched with the stories of a thousand sunrises, broke into wide grins as music, raw and vibrant, spilled from the tiny speaker. A strange calm washed over me. Here they were, with so little, yet their smiles could light up the entire village. I knew they had nothing and I couldn't leave until I learned that happiness isn't about fancy things. It's about finding beauty in the basics. This wasn't about comfort any more. It was about a different kind of education; to find joy in the heart of what truly mattered.

Days blossomed into weeks and the harsh edges of culture shock started to soften. My tongue, once stubbornly resistant to Xitswa, began to pick up a smattering of words, allowing me to have conversations with the villagers and learn more about their lives. The classroom, a dusty haven beneath a sprawling mango tree, became my domain. With chalk scraping across a makeshift blackboard, I became a weaver of knowledge, teaching eager young minds the magic of English and the logic of numbers. Their thirst for learning was a fire that warmed my spirit.

In the afternoons, as the sun dipped below the horizon, painting the sky with vibrant hues, I'd embark on exploratory walks with the other volunteers. Laughter echoed through the village streets as we shared stories – tales woven from unfamiliar customs, surprising encounters, and the slow but steady unravelling of our own preconceived notions. We were sponges, soaking up the wisdom of this vibrant community, learning more about life with every shared meal and every hesitant exchange. Mozambique, once a foreign land to me and my parents, allowed me to have a newfound respect for the resilience of the human spirit.

My initial regret, a bitter pang of fear and culture shock, faded quickly. Running water, a luxury I'd never questioned, became a symbol of my former ignorance. This wasn't just a volunteer experience; it was a humbling revelation. Chibuto wasn't just a village; it was a mirror reflecting the truth – that true happiness wasn't about possessions, but about the connections we forge and the simple joys we learn to appreciate. Mama Veronica and the people of Chibuto became more than just my hosts; they became my teachers, reminding me that the greatest gifts in life are often wrapped in simplicity, kindness and the courage to step outside our comfort zones.

My host mother had the warmest and kindest heart. Her husband had passed away while working in a coal mine in South Africa and out of her four sons, only one of them was alive. Three of her sons had passed away in a car accident. The only son she had left, David, had gone to the capital city, Maputo, to find work. Every meal she prepared, every pot of tea she brewed, overflowed with a silent affection. She saw the fear trembling in my eyes, a fear foreign to her. But with a gentle smile and a language that transcended words, she did everything in her power to weave me into the fabric of her life, to make this stranger a daughter, even if just for a fleeting moment.

My decision to go to Mozambique was the first time in my life where I made a life-changing choice by myself. The voices of doubt, the chorus of 'shoulds' and 'shouldn'ts' that had always hummed in the background, were finally silenced. It was a terrifying yet liberating feeling, a declaration of independence and an act of taking charge of my own future. This wasn't just a trip; it was the beginning of a journey of self-discovery, fuelled by the quiet confidence of finally following my own path.

Bit by bit, I chipped away at the invisible walls that confined the women in my family, and their prescribed futures – marriage, motherhood and domesticity. I craved the freedom to dream beyond the familiar horizon, the courage to carve my own path.

Change rarely arrives on a silver platter; neither is it delivered to our doorsteps. It thrives on those who dare to scratch the itch, who chase the whispers, who aren't afraid to upset the comfortable order of things. The greatest revolutions, the most profound discoveries, all began with a single, nagging question and a tiny seed of curiosity that refuses to be ignored.

Chapter 3

REKINDLED ACTIVISM

15 March 2020: That evening during Nishant's shift after his article went out, I stayed up on my phone desperately reading the latest information on Covid-19. There were reports of our ministers missing emergency meetings, updates on the latest protective equipment guidance by the World Health Organization and data on the urgency to socially distance. Nothing made sense to me; why wasn't any of this being discussed on the news?

I had a very simplistic view of the media at that time. I read headlines and believed every word; I read articles and didn't question their sources of information. Fact-checking, extrapolating data and using my own judgement weren't skills I was equipped with early on. I only identified this blind spot after realising the disparity in my lived experiences and what was being portrayed in the media.

I barely messaged Nishant that night. I didn't want to disturb him in what could have been a shift from hell. Instead, I continued to doom-scroll and absorb all the fear and anxieties that everyone else was facing online at the time. I particularly remember some of my colleagues who were also pregnant, posting photos of their baby bump and their perfectly polished baby nursery. In those fleeting moments, I'd feel a sense of resentment and I would lose my sense of moral clarity. I had to remind myself not to lose sight of what was important at that time; I had a responsibility to support Nishant as his wife in these acute moments.

At this specific point in mid-March, there was one report that had been released by the Royal College of Midwives[1] which stated: 'At present there is one reported case of a woman with Covid-19 who required mechanical ventilation at 30 weeks' gestation, following which she had an emergency caesarean section and made a good recovery.'

In this report, the advice for pregnant women who had been exposed to Covid-19 was to 'self-isolate' and 'stay indoors and avoid contact with others for 14 days'. The guidance even recommended 'not to go to school or NHS settings'.

I was caught in a terrible bind. Choosing the safer option to stay home guaranteed my safety but also felt like a betrayal of my oath to save lives. Taking the risky route of going into work carried the terrible weight of potentially harming myself and my baby. Not only was I worried about getting sick, I was afraid that I wasn't equipped with all the information and data to make a decision. Everything was so new at that time; the evidence on pregnant women especially was just not enough to give me the confidence to continue my job.

After hours of dealing with the aftermath of Nishant's article and dutifully responding to friends and family, I fell asleep. My chest felt heavy with worry that night – I still wasn't sure whether we had done the right thing by speaking up.

The next morning, the baby woke me up with a gentle kick in my womb. I turned over to check my phone; it was only

6am. I hadn't heard from Nishant all night. Usually, he would send me a message joking about how the sandwich I made for him needed more mustard or cheese. Nishant would always look forward to opening his lunchbox and enjoying the selection of sandwiches I had made for him. In fact, now that I look back, there was a time before the pandemic where my main concern about Nishant going into a night shift was what he would eat and if he would get enough rest. Within just a few days, such fatuous worries had transformed into questions of life and death.

I nervously waited for Nishant to walk through the door that morning. Maybe he wouldn't have a job, or worse, a medical licence. As I was getting ready for my 9am shift, my phone was still going off with messages from relatives in India. Many family members were upset that I hadn't told them about my pregnancy. They did not ask how Nishant and I were feeling as doctors on the frontline; they appeared to me blind to the fact that Nishant and I were risking our lives every single day.

I had to switch off from all the noise around me. I had to make that decision for my sanity and for my husband. If I listened to the noise, I knew I would lose focus and I wouldn't be able to provide Nishant with the support he needed.

I wasn't equipped at the time to deal with what was coming my way, but why would I be? I'd never seen or done anything like this before, so how was I supposed to navigate something so unfamiliar? I had rarely heard of stories of South Asian women going against the status quo. Of course, I'd seen plenty of motivational videos on YouTube of women of colour who spoke up for what they believed in, but I never felt any connection with those videos. My circumstances felt completely unique; I was a nobody, fighting a system much bigger than I could imagine.

The only tool I had at that time was having faith in my husband and trusting his instinct.

When Nishant finally walked in, his eyes were as red as I'd ever seen them and I knew he hadn't had any sleep. Usually during night shifts, doctors are encouraged to get some rest when possible. But that night, I knew he wouldn't have had a chance to even think about sleeping. I was too afraid to ask him how his night went. I couldn't just greet him with the usual, 'How was your shift?'

This was different. Nishant wasn't just a junior doctor any more. He was someone who spoke up when nobody else did. He was now seen as a whistleblower.

This is what Nishant said about his shift:

In A&E, I would start my shift at 10pm. I would usually arrive 10–15 minutes earlier for a debrief with the team and to receive a handover from my colleagues who were working throughout the day. Usually, the handover would happen in a dedicated space, where both junior doctors and consultants could sit comfortably and share patients' details and plans. Now, however, things were different. Due to the whole hospital juggling infected spaces and non-infected spaces because of Covid-19, handover was now in a much smaller room, where everybody had to stand up and had no choice but to make eye contact.

At this point, there was no community testing, nor was there adequate staff testing. So, anybody walking through the doors of A&E, including NHS staff, could have been infected with the virus and nobody would ever know. Just before attending handover, I called a colleague of mine to explain this situation. I was looking for some sense of acknowledgement and to some degree, support for my actions. At this point, I was afraid that my article might come across as me trying to spread fear among NHS staff, so I was hoping to get feedback from someone whom I felt was the most level-headed and would give a fair judgement. To my surprise, my colleague felt that the NHS was protecting their staff adequately and everything would be fine. Having this conversation at this specific time, just before entering a room full of my colleagues who had most likely read and judged the article, was far from ideal.

There was a different sort of tension in the room during this handover. It was led by a consultant with whom I had had very little interaction previously and I felt that all eyes were on him. I felt the most anxious I had ever been during my career as a doctor. I was in a heightened state of anxiety – and I felt that nobody was backing me up. I had sent out a clarion call that the British public were about to witness death at a catastrophic scale and all I believed I was receiving was negative reactions.[2, 3, 4]

I have asked Nishant how he felt at this stage and whether he doubted himself or regretted his decisions at any point. He feels he made the right decision, went through the right processes and took this big step after doing a lot of reading and research. There were too many moving parts at the time to confidently predict exactly what would happen over the next few weeks, but there was one big heavy black cloud hanging over him – if he was wrong, he'd look like a fool. He had decided that taking action was the most important step; it was a matter of life and death. He could only worry about the consequences later. There was simply no time to think about the repercussions of his actions because there was a sense of urgency. Every single day where a healthcare worker hadn't been tested or wasn't wearing adequate PPE could have contributed to a tragic death. He had no time to sit and ponder.

Once his handover had finished, the consultant leading the meeting asked Nishant if they could go upstairs and have a quick chat. He said he felt like a lamb about to get slaughtered – it was potentially game over. To his surprise, the consultant was very calm and collected. She didn't get angry or bear any ill-will towards Nishant. She calmly asked if Nishant was okay and if he needed any extra support. The tone of the conversation made Nishant question himself – perhaps he was just overreacting if his seniors thought he needed extra support and help? For those few seconds, Nishant said he thought that maybe he was just taking this all too seriously. That thought was immediately shut down after the consultant said, 'You're more likely to catch the virus in Tesco than you are in hospital.'

That's when he felt that things were wrong. Nishant had done his homework and research. He had stayed up late into the night reading up on papers and trends of the virus as it made its way around the world.

He was confident that his predictions were on track with reality.

* * *

When I started working in the NHS, my introduction to the system was slightly different from most doctors in the UK.

I qualified with a master's in medicine and surgery and so I wasn't obliged to enter an official training programme, which meant that I never received any formal introduction into the NHS.

I had little sense of how I could escalate my concerns. I showed up to work every day and tried to absorb everything like a sponge; I asked lots of questions of my colleagues around me and mostly figured things out as I went along. Thankfully, my colleagues were extremely supportive and understood that as I was trying to learn the ropes of the NHS, I was also trying to emotionally and physically manage a difficult schedule.

The first few months of my job were a relentless emotional rollercoaster. I would face a constant stream of human suffering, from minor ailments to life-or-death situations. The nights left me with dark circles under my eyes, desperate for sleep and warm food. I generally survived on the hospital's snack machine and spent too much of my small salary on cold vending machine sandwiches and snicker bars. The days were just as bad, except that some days, I would be able to see the sun shine through the windows and that was always a gentle reminder that I was still fortunate to have a life outside the hospital.

Some of my patients were destined to die in hospital. They woke up every morning with the hope that their medical situation might improve and they would be able to go back home to their family. Some were too weak to be transferred home and some would have drastic turns overnight. As I documented the time of death of my patients, the line between healer and witness blurred. It always left me wondering: was this all there was in life, this constant fight against the inevitable?

I always tried to have a sense of perspective, but at the end of the day, we're all humans. I knew I needed support and I so desperately wished I had a senior colleague to raise even the smallest of my concerns to – but I genuinely believed that we just had to get on with it. I wouldn't dare complain or make it seem as if I was being difficult. Speaking up could have jeopardised my job and, subsequently, my career.

I wouldn't dare take any action that could throw away my six years of hard work in medical school. Getting to the stage of working as a doctor in the NHS involved too much sacrifice, financial risk and, most importantly, time. I had dedicated my whole life to working towards this position, as had my parents. I wouldn't dream of throwing it all away.

There was a similar fear looming over me and my colleagues in March 2020. We were told that everything was under control and that if we were concerned about patient safety, we could let our seniors know. The only problem here was I was not aware of the protocol for how we could escalate our concerns. If others were similarly not aware then this could be crucial when it came to patient and staff safety. During the early days of the pandemic, we all expected a few teething problems, but it really just felt that mistakes were happening in front of us and we did not do enough to address them. The immediate consequence of this was, in my view, more suffering and perhaps even more deaths.

In early March, the World Health Organization had released guidance on rationalising use of PPE. The guidance clearly predicted that countries around the world would hit a shortage of PPE gear due to a backlog in the global supply chain. At that time, the guidance was to remove and safely dispose of PPE after close contact with a Covid-19 patient and don a new set of PPE gear (which included masks) for the next patient.

We had patients walking through the doors of A&E who weren't tested in the community, so we would examine them blindly with only our masks, because technically they weren't positive until proven otherwise. If they happened to be positive, we would then use those same masks to see the next patient. This practice was incredibly unsafe, yet, whenever I asked for a new mask, I was silenced into accepting that I just had to continue with what I was given.

I and many of my colleagues were penalised for picking up a new mask after every patient. I had nurses come to me in tears, begging me to find a way to help them use new masks. They were concerned that if they caught the virus and went back home to their elderly parents, they would make them ill. The knock-on effect of the crisis that hit healthcare workers has been underestimated to this day. Nishant and I lived on separate floors for six months to protect each other and our baby. These sacrifices didn't feel like a burden on us at the time – we genuinely felt that it was our duty to put our patients and the British public first.

Many of us felt uncomfortable with the unreasonable PPE guidelines and how some of our concerns were being managed. The biggest question hanging over all of us was, 'Where do we go from here? Where do we go if our managers and our consultants cannot help us?' This was a matter of patient safety. If, as doctors, we didn't feel protected, where did that leave our patients?

Nishant's article ignited a firestorm of silent nods and passionate rebuttals among our colleagues. It left me baffled – how could something so clear to me be so murky for others?

I cannot help feeling that part of the answer was that many of our colleagues were Black, Asian, and Minority Ethnic (BAME) immigrants. Many of them carried the weight of a hard-won life, a dream of a new beginning in the UK. Putting their heads down and powering through disagreements was the price they'd paid. In their eyes, it just wasn't worth the risk. Staying silent was the safest option.

The virus snatched so many, including a colleague's relatives, dragging them into the sterile purgatory of the intensive care unit. FaceTime calls offered a flimsy lifeline, their voices muffled by the hiss of oxygen masks. She lost two close relatives in quick succession. The goodbyes, if there were any, were stolen whispers through an iPad. They died alone, their final breaths without much comfort. She had her own grief to contend with alongside long shifts – a chilling reminder of the price many healthcare workers paid.

This is just one story of a family who suffered unnecessarily.

This multiplied at an exponential rate as the weeks went on. I started to see my own colleagues, who I was close to, end up on ventilators; consultants who had spent their lives devoted and dedicated to the NHS became unwell, yet our politicians were telling us that everything was under control in the daily press briefings.

I remember one instance where a Sky News reporter had mentioned that they were considering setting up burials in the middle of big cities such as London.[5] I paused the TV, went back to double check I hadn't misheard what the reporter had said. The government was coordinating plans to create a network of temporary mortuaries to cope with the rising death toll.

How were we, as a nation, simply expected to accept this? My helplessness soon festered into righteous anger – an anger that gave me an itch to go out and make a change. I wasn't able to sit still. I couldn't just sit back and watch. If I was complicit, it made me no better than the same politicians who were moving our country towards a disaster.

* * *

Evidence was collated by the Doctors' Association UK, which found that doctors and nurses were being warned by hospital and other NHS bodies not to raise their concerns publicly.[6]

Dr Samantha Batt Rawden, Doctors' Association UK's president, said:

> *At this time when we desperately need every single doctor on the frontline, some have had their careers threatened, and at least two doctors have been sent home from work. This is unacceptable. Doctors have a moral duty to make their concerns regarding Covid-19 public if these cannot be resolved locally.*

The reality of what NHS workers were facing was seen on social media by thousands if not millions of people. Nurses in bin bags, doctors wearing science goggles to see patients confirmed with coronavirus, it was all the evidence our politicians didn't want the public to see. The same people who were telling healthcare workers not to speak up were often sitting in their offices far away from infected wards and departments, making these decisions. In fact, some of them were even working from home. What did they know about our experiences?

The only tool I had at that time was my voice. I had to channel all this frustration and energy and try to have a positive impact where I could. It was the least I could do.

Unlike my husband, I felt that I had to remain anonymous. I was worried that if I did get into trouble, it could affect my maternity leave pay and any future possibility of getting my job back after giving birth.

Of course, at that time, I wished I could get a megaphone and scream from the rooftops that we were in great trouble, but I knew that wouldn't help anyone and it wouldn't change anything. So, I decided to take small steps. Small acts that would hopefully soften the blow of this crisis on NHS staff.

* * *

In 2009, the Healthcare Commission, the regulator of NHS care standards at the time, published a report on the care provided at Stafford Hospital.[7] The report found that the hospital had a 'serious culture of neglect' and that patients had been 'left to suffer unnecessarily'. The report also found that staff were 'overworked and demoralised' and that there was a 'lack of leadership' at the hospital.

The report's findings led to a public inquiry, chaired by Robert Francis QC. The inquiry heard evidence from patients, families, staff and managers. The inquiry's report,[8] published in 2013, found that there had been 'a catastrophic failure of care' at Stafford Hospital. It also found that there had been 'a culture of denial' at the hospital and that there had been 'a failure of leadership' (p.3).

The inquiry's report led to a number of changes at Stafford Hospital. The hospital was placed in special measures and a new management team was appointed. A large amount of funding was allocated to improve the hospital's facilities and services.

The Stafford Hospital scandal had a significant impact on the NHS and led to a number of changes in the way that the NHS is regulated and monitored. It also led to a greater focus on patient safety and quality of care.

The Stafford Hospital scandal is a reminder that even in the world's most advanced healthcare systems, patients can be harmed if they do not receive the care that they need. It is also a reminder that the NHS is only as good as the people who work in it. If staff are overworked and demoralised, patients will suffer.

This independent inquiry stated that hospital patients had been left 'sobbing and humiliated' by uncaring staff: 'This is a story of appalling and unnecessary suffering of hundreds of people.' 'They were failed by a system which ignored the warning signs and put corporate self-interest and cost control ahead of patients and their safety.'

To my surprise, this 200-page report goes into the granular detail as to how the NHS can and should help healthcare workers speak up. It works towards creating the right environments to report any issues they feel may be affecting patient safety.

In March 2020, I had not read this report. We've had numerous occasions as junior doctors where we've had teaching days during our working hours. We've spent hours learning about human anatomy and physiology and put in a great deal of effort to stay up to date with our medical knowledge. But all of this feels futile if we're simply not educated on how we can put our patients first. After all, that's the crux of our job. We work for our patients and their safety.

More education on learning how to centre our work around this can create a great difference in our care for patients within the NHS. We should invest more time in presenting cases such as the Stafford Hospital case to juniors and reflecting on how we can all work towards creating a safer environment where we can raise concerns and, in turn, help our patients.

Of almost 20,000 NHS staff members included in the 2013 survey, 30 per cent who had raised a concern had felt unsafe afterwards. This independent inquiry was asked to consider what further action was necessary to protect health service staff who speak out in the public interest, with the ultimate aim of creating an 'open and honest reporting culture in the NHS'.

Sir Robert Francis had stated in an interview: 'Failure to speak up can cost lives. I began this review with an open mind about whether there are things getting in the way of NHS staff speaking up.'[9]

However, the evidence received by the inquiry confirmed that there is a serious issue within the NHS. This issue is not just about whistleblowing – it is fundamentally a safety issue.

Ultimately, all of this can only be achieved if the voices and opinions of healthcare workers are acknowledged and if we are encouraged to speak up any time we are concerned.

The term whistleblowing makes people uncomfortable. Whistleblowing is a controversial issue. Some people believe that whistleblowers are heroes who are willing to risk their careers and reputations to expose wrongdoing. Others believe that whistleblowers are troublemakers who are more interested in self-promotion than in helping others.

In the UK, whistleblowing is protected by law. The Public

Interest Disclosure Act 1998 (PIDA) protects employees who raise concerns about wrongdoing in the workplace. The PIDA also protects employees who make disclosures to the media or to other organisations.

The term 'whistleblower' is thought to have originated in the 19th century, when railway engineers would blow whistles to warn of oncoming trains. In the early 20th century, the term was used to describe people who blew the whistle on corruption in government and business.

The history of whistleblowing in the NHS is a long and complex one. However, it is clear that whistleblowers have played a vital role in improving patient safety and raising standards of care. The introduction of new legislation and guidance has helped to protect whistleblowers and has created a more open and transparent culture in the NHS.

Despite these reforms, there is still more that needs to be done to protect whistleblowers in the NHS. People should be able to raise concerns without fear of reprisal, and they should be supported by their employers and colleagues. The NHS needs to create a culture where whistleblowing is seen as a positive thing, not a negative one.

The word 'whistleblower' hung in the air after Nishant's article came out, a label often shrouded in negativity. Yet, I didn't see him as a troublemaker, but a sculptor chipping away at a broken system. If being a whistleblower meant standing on the side of truth, even if it meant facing the winds of adversity, then so be it. Nishant's bravery ignited a spark within me – a reminder that sometimes the most valuable things in life are not attained by comfort, but by the courage to disrupt it.

Chapter 4

SMALL STEPS

The carefully curated image, the one of unwavering resolve and boundless resources, began to crumble on social media. Healthcare workers were posting selfies with their faces etched with red marks from wearing tight masks. This was the truth. Unfiltered and raw. A stark difference to the sanitised narratives coming from our ministers' offices. This wasn't the narrative spun by those in power, a narrative devoid of discomfort and sacrifice.

Frustration was roiling within me for weeks, fuelling me with a desperate need to act. The only weapon I had with me was my voice. Nishant saw the world in stark black and white, and was ready to shout the truth from the rooftops. But I had the weight of an impending birth pressing down. I had a fear of retribution, of lost maternity pay, of a future career hanging by a thread. Watching as a bystander in this unfolding crisis wasn't an option for me. So, I made a choice. Small acts, I decided, were the weapons I'd use, each one a tiny contribution, chipping away at the mountain of challenges faced by the NHS. It was a long road ahead, but sometimes, the smallest steps lead to the greatest journeys.

My close friend, Manjit Gill MBE, was working on her

charity, Binti International, at the time. She set up the charity to improve education on women's health, hygiene and periods. Manjit is based in Weybridge, Surrey, and through the help of a community of elderly ladies in her local village, they were working on a big project to sew and distribute reusable sanitary products.

When lockdown hit us, Manjit wanted to help her team of elderly ladies stay active and find purpose in their daily routine. A lot of her work involved travelling across the country to give talks and set up distribution points to deliver free sanitary products for women. In March 2020, Manjit realised that she had to pivot. With lockdown, all her travels and workshops came to a halt. So, she started to work on ideas to help healthcare workers get through the pandemic.

Whiteley Village is a retirement village in Weybridge. Manjit and her team had set up a sewing club there where the ladies created Binti Period Bags. These bags were donated to schools and food banks to assist with the distribution of free menstrual products. It was a fun, weekly group designed for the women to get together, have a natter and support a local charity to provide a sustainable solution for providing menstrual products.

In March 2020, some businesses in the UK exploited the shortage of surgical masks during the Covid-19 pandemic. Some businesses raised the prices of surgical masks significantly, even though the cost of production had not increased. Some hoarded surgical masks in an effort to drive up prices. This made it even more difficult for people to obtain the masks they needed. There were even some businesses which sold counterfeit surgical masks, and this put people at risk of infection.

So when Manjit called me one day for our usual catch up, we came up with the idea of creating a project where we could ask our team of elderly ladies to knit and sew homemade masks. Of course, at that time, we knew that surgical masks were the optimal choice for protection. The desperate scramble for masks had created a black market out of pharmacies. Surgical masks became rare diamonds and only added to the anxiety of the pandemic. We knew that we would all suffer from being locked inside and our only saving grace was leaving the house safely with a protective mask.

We thought that if we could provide the public with masks that are washable and reusable, perhaps it would spread a sense of calm and confidence when they decided to venture out to the supermarket or local shops.

Manjit has always been a woman to fight her way through any barrier faced in front of her. Setting up Binti International came with so many challenges, especially when trying to educate women from South Asian backgrounds about periods and remove the stigma around them in orthodox communities. When we came up with this idea, Manjit immediately created an online document with details of inventory, materials and delivery methods. Any profits made from our mask project would go towards the charity and contribute to the important work of Binti International.

This conversation unlocked a door to a new kind of action, one that wasn't bound by red tape. It created a fire in my belly and finally I could feel my anger slowly turn into determination and hope. Although I was still working in the hospital and helping with the coronavirus crisis, I felt stuck within a system. I felt stifled by protocols, guidelines and rules. Now, I felt a new sense of freedom. I would knock on my neighbours' doors with my Binti masks and see the smiles on their faces. I would do regular check-ins with my neighbours and they would express their gratitude; they would feel a little less lonely and some small chat was a welcome change from the ongoing situation.

Within a few days, I went from delivering bad news to patients and relatives during my hospital shifts, to delivering masks to friends and family in the evening. Nishant constantly reminded me to slow down and rest my pregnant body. But with Manjit by my side, there was a strange solace, a balm to the relentless worry. Working alongside Manjit on our shared mission was a way to channel the storm brewing inside me into something productive.

Our mask project started to gain momentum. We were getting emails and orders for our masks and our community of elderly ladies in the village were finding so much joy in making the masks, despite being locked down.

Nishant was doing a few interviews dotted around his very busy A&E shifts around this time, but he still tried to keep a low profile as he felt that his article in *The Guardian* had not gone down well with some of his colleagues and seniors. As I started to open up more and find my voice, there was a palpable energy in our house. Our combined determination to make things right was growing every day.

What if we joined hands and combined our fire? How much more of an impact could we have if we worked together? We soon found out that we could change the course of an entire system together.

* * *

One morning, I received an Instagram message from a news outlet in India. I had been following them for a while and they had asked me if I could get involved in one of the pieces they were working on related to healthcare workers and Covid-19. This was the first time a journalist had contacted me personally during the pandemic and I wasn't sure if it would be safe to engage.

I was sitting in the staff room in the oncology ward where I was placed at that time. Patients were waiting for life-saving chemotherapy but we just didn't know how and when their treatments would take place. There were talks of sending them home and delaying treatments and turning the ward into an acute ward with Covid-19 patients. This eventually did happen, but I genuinely never believed it would. To some extent, I was still in denial, mostly out of fear.

I felt I was walking on a moral tightrope. How could we turn our backs on the patients who entrusted their very lives to our hands? We had to make difficult phone calls to patients and their families explaining that we had to delay treatment until we felt it was safe for them to leave their homes and for them to come back into hospitals. These conversations left me in tears every time. There was nothing in medical school or my time as a junior doctor which had prepared me for this.

As I was reading the message from the journalist in India, a nurse had walked in and burst into tears. She took her mask off, and I could see the indentation of the mask on her skin which she had been wearing all day.

'I'm fed up with not knowing what's going to happen. Every patient I speak to is worried their cancer will kill them before the virus.' Her voice was trembling and she felt helpless. Nobody had any answers at this stage; we were all trying our best and complying with the rules from above.

I gave her a glass of water and put my hand on her shoulder. I couldn't give her a hug as we were told to avoid close contact and because of my pregnancy, I was extra cautious.

This was the moment I realised that there was no coverage in the media on what was happening inside hospitals. The sanitised pronouncements filtering through television screens felt like a cruel mockery of our reality. The human cost, the raw desperation, the dance with death we performed every shift – these were absent from the nightly news. It was a world unseen, unheard, a truth shrouded by statistics and empty platitudes. We were fighting a desperate battle, and the outside world remained blissfully unaware.

Nobody had seen images or videos of nurses crying into their mask, of doctors trying to console their colleagues or of healthcare workers donning inadequate PPE to see their patients. Without this imagery, it was impossible for the public to have a real idea of what was going on. We could show up in the media as much as we wanted and try and verbalise how we felt and explain ourselves, but it wouldn't paint a fair picture of the raw reality. We yearned for the public to see – truly see – the unvarnished reality behind the heroism.

I wondered if this disconnect, this chasm between the lived experience and the televised narrative, wasn't the very reason our esteemed leadership so tragically misread the situation.

I went back to read my message from the journalist and she had specifically asked if I could make a short vlog-style film about what it was like to be working inside the hospital. Of course, at the time, the pressing issue was the inadequate

PPE supply, and the guidelines which were changing frequently. I innocently suggested I make a short video on what it was like to prepare to see a Covid-19 patient and the equipment involved – mainly to emphasise the absurdity of wearing a plastic apron and, in some cases, school-donated science goggles to see a patient.

My suggestion was a knee-jerk reaction. The world had to witness this – the indignity, the helplessness. We were suffering, invisible beneath flimsy masks and ill-fitting gowns. We deserved better, deserved to be seen as more than expendable pawns.

I knew I couldn't film this at home; it had to be done in the hospital where I had access to the equipment. Before agreeing to do this, I'd meticulously drafted the video script; a desperate plea for help disguised as a national emergency. I thought I was playing it safe by making a generalised video. But unfortunately, my naivety left me with another shock.

Looking back now with the knowledge I have acquired over the last three years, I feel that the journalists did what I asked which was not to name the place where I worked. They respected my situation and agreed to all the edits I had suggested. They released this piece in good faith as they wanted to raise the headlines with regards to the mismanagement of doctors in the UK working on the frontline, including those who were from ethnic minority groups like India.

Before I sent the video to the editor, I wanted to talk it through with Nishant. He'd already been through so much emotional stress, I wasn't sure if this would be the right move. I trusted Nishant's judgement and supported him with every decision he made. I knew he could separate his emotions and think with much greater clarity than I could. But I had no time, the editors were pressed on a deadline and Nishant was so busy in A&E, I didn't want to bother him.

My gut feeling told me to just send it and deal with the consequences later. After a few messages back and forth between the editors to cut out, blur and edit a few things that could possibly give away the hospital I was working at, we came to the final cut. I was so particular with the editing that even if a shelf had a label with the acronym of the hospital in the tiniest font, I asked if that could be blurred out. I was so paranoid that someone would zoom in and discover where I was that I became obsessed with the tiniest of details.

Ultimately, the journalists were just as determined as I was to get this story out, so they adhered to my instructions and very patiently followed my detailed feedback.

The next day, I opened up Instagram and there it was. The moment I was hoping for and dreading at the same time. Over 500 notifications and countless direct messages (DMs) popped up on my screen. I knew the video was out, but I was too nervous to even open the video, read the comments and check the notifications. This is what I was trying to achieve in the first place – an awakening from the public, both online and offline, to the reality of what doctors were facing, but the slightly uncomfortable thing was that it had my face and my name on it.

'Dr Meenal Viz exposes the reality of doctors abroad.' It sounded like a sensational headline, but at this point, it had to be done this way. The headlines had evoked some urgency, even if it looked dramatised. I closed the app, put my phone away and went back into work pretending I had seen nothing. I was too afraid to deal with the consequences now, but perhaps it was too late. Some damage had already been done.

As I was finishing my ward round, I received a phone call from my consultant. He was the clinical director of the oncology unit and pretty much ran the whole department. He was always kind and considerate towards his juniors; he never took us for granted and I always felt comfortable raising concerns with him. He was affable, respected within the hospital and was very determined to offer the best support and care for his patients. When he had initially offered me the job, I loved learning from him. He had a very special way of communicating with his patients and making sure they were happy with his plans and treatments. Even in the face of death, all his family meetings would end in smiles – a unique skill which takes years of hard work and effort to master.

'Oh, hi Meenal, just a quick thing. I'm literally being wheeled into theatre for my back surgery right now but I just wanted to have a quick chat with you. I've been informed of a video that's been released online and the Trust aren't very happy about it. I know you haven't mentioned anything against us and you're working very hard, but can you please make sure that's removed from the internet.'

My legs started shaking underneath me and my lips started quivering for a minute. I paused and my brain went through all the scenes I had witnessed; the nurses crying, me and my husband living on separate floors, my colleagues coming out of Covid wards with mask indentations on their faces.

I snapped back and thought to myself, 'No, I won't accept this. We are suffering and instead of helping us, you are effectively silencing us.'

After a few moments of collecting my thoughts and trying to formulate a measured response, I replied, 'I hope you understand this is not about the Trust, nor is it a personal attack on you or your department. I have no intention of damaging the reputation of this Trust, but I do believe my experiences as a junior doctor during the pandemic need to be acknowledged.'

The response I received was that if such a situation were to occur again, there might be consequences, though the request to take down the video was not explicitly repeated. Reluctantly, I chose to leave it at that. I did not take action regarding the video and allowed it to spread unchecked online.

As the video was making its rounds on the internet, I was receiving messages from doctors across the world. They felt helpless against the enormity of the virus. Doctors in India, especially, had seen my video and they were telling me how they were receiving abuse from the public because some people felt doctors weren't doing enough to save the lives of patients. The reality was that we were doing everything we could and beyond that – we just didn't have the tools to provide the best care. We were sent into war with a butter knife.

I started to walk around the hospital with my head down. I didn't want to bump into anyone or make eye contact. A part of me felt shame. I felt that I was deceiving my colleagues and bosses by exposing the truth.

I went back to my ward and continued as usual with my work and again, I received another call. Receiving phone calls from unknown numbers is particularly scary, especially when you know you've done something that might get you into trouble! My heart started racing again. What if this time it was a senior boss or a more serious warning from above? I was tempted to ignore the call and already planned my excuse if I received a follow-up call or email – I was too busy dealing with sick patients and the chaos of the virus.

That was the easy option. But taking the path of least resistance wouldn't do me, or my patients, any good and I knew that deep down, this was all on me. I'd made the decision to make the video and I agreed to put it online. I could have erased everything within a few minutes, but that would mean erasing the truth and, subsequently, erasing history.

I stood up, took a deep breath and answered the call.

'Oh hi, Dr Viz, I'm calling from the comms team. I was just checking in to see how you were doing?'

I thought this was very odd. A non-threatening, calm and seemingly kind voice was on the other end of the phone.

'I'm fine, thank you.'

'So I'm just calling as we've seen that you've been speaking to a few journalists about the pandemic and the Trust isn't too happy about this. I hope you understand.'

I had no idea who this person was. I had no idea what power they held within the Trust and I also had no idea where she was.

'Sure, thanks for the call. But I hope you understand that I am purely trying to voice the struggles we are facing as doctors within the NHS at this time. I have never mentioned which hospital I work at, nor have I mentioned any names. I have kept everything under the radar.'

There was a sudden silence and I couldn't hear anything from the other side for a few minutes.

I patiently waited and walked up and down the corridor waiting for a response.

'Oh sorry, Dr Viz, we just got a surprise delivery of pizza from the community to say thank you to all the staff who've been working hard during this crisis.'

Doctors, nurses, techs – all of us on the frontlines – were pleading for reinforcements, for the most basic tools to shield ourselves from the virus. On the top floor of our hospitals sat, among others, the communications managers. But it felt as if they were not advocating for us. It was a bitter pill to swallow.

'Enjoy! I have a very busy ward; I need to get back to work. Thank you for your call.'

I hung up and decided not to entertain any more of this.

I kept the video online and surprisingly, didn't receive any more phone calls.

Talking to consultants and managers used to fill me with dread. But now, as I walked into their offices, my chin was held a little higher, my shoulders squared. The questions I once timidly mumbled were now delivered with a clear, unwavering tone. The anger that had simmered within me was morphing, transforming into a potent cocktail of courage and conviction. It fuelled my every word, every rebuttal, every demand. With each interaction, I felt a shift within. I wasn't the same person I was a few weeks ago.

One thing was certain – I was no longer afraid. I was ready to fight, for myself, for my colleagues, for what was right. With every step I took, with every voice I raised, I felt myself becoming someone entirely new. Someone strong, fearless and utterly unstoppable.

* * *

As the pandemic progressed, consultant doctors continued to play a leading role in providing care to patients with Covid-19 and also helped to develop new treatments and procedures for managing the virus. Days that were once filled with meticulously planned surgeries and specialist clinics morphed into a desperate scramble to keep pace with the relentless influx.

In the early phase of the pandemic, many consultants stepped up courageously, leading their teams on the frontlines and supporting junior colleagues in difficult circumstances. This was a humbling display of leadership. However, as the situation evolved and the risk of infection grew, some consultants who were vulnerable or at higher risk moved to working from home. While this was necessary to protect their health, it also meant that junior doctors, including myself and my husband, often faced increased exposure and responsibility, highlighting the challenges of maintaining fairness and support during an unprecedented crisis.

In contrast, consultants in other departments, such as surgery and oncology, faced a different reality. With patient admissions restricted due to infection control measures, these consultants were able to work remotely, distanced from the daily turmoil of the hospital. The disparity in their experiences was stark, as some were insulated from the crisis while others were thrust into its centre.

* * *

The first whispers of Dr Li Wenliang's story began swirling through social media. This young ophthalmologist, barely older than some of our colleagues, was one of the first voices to raise the alarm about a mysterious new virus in Wuhan in December 2019. In a private chat with fellow doctors, he shared concerns about patients exhibiting SARS-like symptoms and urged them to take precautions. His warnings were not met with acknowledgement or action but were instead suppressed. Chinese authorities accused him of spreading 'false rumours', and forced him to sign a statement of reprimand.[1] Within weeks, the virus he tried to warn others about swept through Wuhan. Tragically, Dr Li contracted Covid-19 while treating an infected patient and died on 7 February 2020, at just 33 years old.

Dr Li became a symbol, a testament to the precarious tightrope we all walked. His tragic death, leaving behind a young family, cast a long shadow, a stark reminder of the human cost of silenced truth. His story struck a chord with me. Like Nishant, he was a young doctor, trying to protect everyone around him. It resonated too painfully with Nishant's story and that terrified me. Dr Li's story became a grim mirror reflecting our own hypocrisy.

Here we were, turning a blind eye to the very same injustice unfolding in our own backyard.

Meanwhile, my own video, a raw and desperate plea for proper PPE, found its way into the hands of doctors across the globe. A chorus of helplessness echoed back, messages from India painting a picture of doctors facing not just a deadly virus, but public abuse as well. The frustration was palpable, a shared burden across continents. We were the ones staring death in the face every day, the ones sacrificing our own safety for the sake of others. Dr Li's story became a beacon, a reminder that even in the face of immense pressure, some voices refuse to be silenced. And my own small act, a desperate plea for help, had somehow managed to spark a global conversation – a testament to the power of solidarity in the face of a crisis.

Chapter 5

MARY'S DEATH AND ITS FALLOUT

13 April 2020: Nishant shuffled through the door at 8.30am after his night shift. I was packing my bag, getting ready for work as he walked in. Something felt different. His eyes showed a deeper kind of weariness, a soul-sucking exhaustion that spoke of a different kind of battle. The smile that usually played on his lips, a beacon of warmth and resilience, was absent that morning. It wasn't just fatigue clinging to him, the kind that lingered after a particularly gruelling shift in the Covid ward. This was a deeper exhaustion, the kind that makes you question your own existence.

A cold dread bloomed in my gut. This wasn't another reprimand from a tone-deaf manager or a frustrated colleague. This was something bigger. We were tightrope walkers in a hurricane, and the ground seemed to be rapidly disappearing. Fear was a constant companion these days, but this was a fear tinged with a new, horrifying possibility.

The words, 'You all right?' got caught in my throat. The defiance that usually flickered in his eyes, the same defiance that had got us both through countless late nights and relentless waves of the pandemic, was extinguished.

'Don't worry about it. Go to work. We'll talk later.' But in his gaze was a silent plea for a burden to be shared, a weight too heavy for him to bear alone.

'Nishant, are you sure you're okay? Maybe I should stay at home today? You've been through a lot these past few weeks. Let me help.'

Nishant knew my offer was genuine, the least I could do for the man who'd become my anchor in this storm. I was desperate to stay and offer him the comfort he needed. But I knew he needed to be alone to process the last 12 hours of his shift and I had to respect that. I left for work that morning with a heavy burden on my shoulders. Nishant wasn't alone; it was a battle we were facing together.

The exhaustion that clung to me after my shift was a familiar weight, a backpack filled with the day's anxieties and triumphs. As I stepped into our home, I noticed Nishant was sitting on the living room floor with his back against the sofa, his posture a crumpled tapestry of despair. He had his phone on the coffee table with his speakerphone on. All I could hear was an unfamiliar voice spewing forth a torrent of emotions – anger, raw and rasping, punctuated by choked sobs.

He listened intently. Each 'Okay, calm down' he offered sounded less like reassurance and more like a mantra he repeated to himself, a desperate attempt to maintain his own equilibrium. The words 'one thing at a time' tumbled from his lips every so often as he tried to keep up with the conversation.

The familiar warmth of our apartment was absent and an unsettling silence hung heavy in the air. As I walked into the kitchen, his breakfast was untouched and the lunch I'd lovingly packed remained tightly wrapped. Even the sink held a single glass – he hadn't eaten or had anything to drink all day. I felt that Nishant, my pillar of strength, was starting to crumble under an unseen weight.

I continued with my usual routine after work – shower, wash my clothes and disinfect my equipment. As I stepped out of the shower, I ran a hand over my reflection in the fogged-up mirror. The familiar contours of my body were subtly changing. My once-rounded belly button had receded, replaced by a smooth indentation, and the soft skin around my waist was starting to stretch. It was a beautiful change, a sign of the miracle growing inside me, yet an unsettling tremor ran through me.

Would this tiny flicker of life inside me ever get a chance to meet the sunshine, to feel the warmth of the world beyond these walls?

Yet, looking at the reflection again, I saw not just the worry, but a fierce determination. This wasn't just about survival; it was about holding on to hope, about bringing a new life into a world that desperately needed light.

I came back into the living room and Nishant had just finished his very intense phone call. Again, I was very gentle in asking Nishant anything at this point. He was sleep deprived and I knew he was dealing with a very sensitive situation.

'Nishant, is everything okay? Is there anything I can do to help?'

'Meenal, you won't believe what happened. I haven't slept all day and I haven't eaten.'

'I know, I can see. What's actually happened?'

'A pregnant nurse, Mary Agyapong, passed away at the

hospital last night. I just spoke to one of her colleagues and she was explaining what had happened.'

'And what about her baby?'

'The baby is in the neonatal intensive care unit. Her husband lives down the road from us and he hasn't been able to visit the baby because of Covid-19 restrictions.'

This nurse, a beacon of hope for many of her patients, wasn't just another name on a news report. She was a woman who, like me, had cradled a dream beneath her own heart. Just moments ago, my fingers were caressing my belly, praying for our safety and the protection of our family.

'She also left behind her two-year-old son.'

Nishant never came upstairs that night to say goodnight. He crashed on the sofa with his phone on his chest.

He was up for almost 40 hours at this point. He was running on fumes.

* * *

Two months before I was due to give birth, Nishant and I received a WhatsApp message from Ernest, Mary's husband. He sent us an invitation to Mary's funeral and wanted us both to be there. The faceless statistics, the newsreel blurbs of loss – they all solidified into a painful reality. Here was a name, a life cut short, a family left with a hollow echo of laughter and love. But a familiar knot formed in my stomach. How would I explain this to my family? Telling them that at 32 weeks pregnant, I was attending a funeral.

In the Hindu culture, attending funerals during a pregnancy is seen as a bad omen. Even whispering the word 'death' was said to attract ill winds, potentially harming the unborn child. Now here I was again, trying to help and support a family and at the same time, formulating a satisfactory explanation for my mother who would call me asking me why I thought going to this funeral was a good idea.

The weight of tradition, a suffocating cloak woven from 'should' and 'supposed to', pressed down on me. Each stolen moment of introspection chipped away at my spirit. I craved a life unburdened by the constant need to justify my actions.

When we arrived at the funeral, Nishant asked me if I wanted to stay in the car. He was worried that the ceremony might be too overwhelming for me. As I stepped out of the car, I looked at him and gave him the same look of determination as I did when I went out to protest. My hands were shaking and my heart started racing. From a distance, I could hear women wailing in desperation, asking God to bring Mary back.

As we walked towards them, tears were rolling down my cheeks and Nishant squeezed my hand to remind me that again, no matter how difficult a situation may seem to us, we would always get through it together.

At the entrance to the funeral, I could see everyone congregating around the priest. We were all asked to keep the usual one metre distance from one another as per the government guidelines, which made it difficult to console anyone or even offer a hug to anybody who was grieving that morning. Throughout the funeral, we were all consoling each other through eye contact. Looking at each other with the same feeling of hopelessness – we had lost a precious soul and nobody was there to protect her when she needed it the most. Now, here we were at her funeral and there was absolutely nothing we could do or say to make Ernest feel better or bring the mother of his children back to this world.

Before the funeral, I wasn't aware that Mary's father had also passed away with Covid-19 at another hospital. The funeral was dedicated to both Mary and her father. As I stood outside among all the mourners who came to pay their respects, I had images of news headlines and media interviews of Matt Hancock proudly boasting about the PPE he had procured for the NHS. How could we stand here, mourning the loss of loved ones, while those who promised to protect us revelled in self-serving narratives?

While I've been writing this book, the news of the 'Partygate' scandal has been revealed. It is a classic example of the hypocrisy and corruption that has come to define British politics. While the rest of the country was suffering under a harsh lockdown, the Prime Minister and his cronies were partying at Downing Street.

During the early stages of the pandemic, many were attending funerals of their loved ones online, through Zoom. The pandemic had completely changed the way we grieve. We couldn't hold our loved ones close to us, nor could we kiss them goodbye. The intimacy we all desperately needed to get through the most difficult times was robbed from us by the virus.

As I was going through these images in my head like a camera roll, I could hear the wailing and screaming of all those who loved Mary so dearly. A few days before the funeral, I remember learning about the NHS and Social Care Coronavirus Life Assurance Scheme, set up in April 2020 to provide financial support to the families of NHS and social care workers who died from Covid-19. It offered a lump sum payment of £60,000, not subject to tax.

My stomach churned at the thought that our government

felt it could 'pay off' its mistakes. There is no amount of money that can heal the wounds of losing a loved one. I was also horrified to learn that this scheme came with a few conditions. One of them was that the family had to agree to release the government from any liability for their loss.

As of March 2023, around 760 claims had been lodged under the scheme and 732 payments had been made. However, it is estimated that around 2000 NHS and social care workers died from Covid-19 during the pandemic, so it is likely that many families are still waiting to receive a payment or did not apply.

Two coffins were lowered into the ground that morning. Inside one coffin was a dedicated nurse, mother and wife who never got to hold her newborn baby. In the other was her father, who would have never dreamed of being buried on the same day as his daughter.

Chapter 6

TO PROTEST OR NOT TO PROTEST

A Moral Dilemma

'Meenal, I think we need to protest.'

Nishant scrolled through a relentless tide of articles echoing the desperation of doctors. But amid the cacophony, something felt deafeningly silent. There was no image, no singular beacon that captured the spirit of our profession.

Nishant felt that the world needed to see a doctor, not just another statistic, but a symbol of unwavering resistance. Someone who stood tall, a figure radiating a fierce determination and a testament to the unwavering spirit of the medical profession. Nishant was determined to bring down the systems silencing us – the systems more concerned with procedure than protection.

I agreed immediately, but I felt my stomach churn. I understood the fierce fire in his eyes, the desperate need to scream the truth from the rooftops. But our past experiences had taught us some very important lessons. We could not help feeling that the lack of support from some of our superiors indicated a preference for docile silence, a well-oiled machine of obedience. Although our jobs weren't threatened, we still felt on edge from Nishant's collaboration with Carole, that explosive article exposing the cracks in the system. My own video hadn't exactly garnered any praise from the powers above me either.

The consequences loomed large, but the alternative – burying our concerns under a mountain of complicit silence – felt even heavier. The decision hung in the air, a pregnant pause filled with the unspoken weight of rebellion. Maybe, just maybe, silence wasn't the only answer to our suffering.

We were still in very strict lockdown. Only the most essential journeys were permitted. Was a protest classified as essential travel?

The decision to protest was unnerving, but also ignited an ember of hope. Could one tiny act of defiance truly make a difference?

The days after Mary's death blurred as Nishant and I exchanged ideas while we were at work. Nishant meticulously dissected his contract with Health Education England, reminding me to search through mine. Every clause, every comma, was scrutinised in a desperate attempt to armour ourselves against any retribution.

That week, I had my oral glucose tolerance test, a standard procedure for any pregnant woman during pregnancy. The appointment took a few hours, which gave me plenty of time and space to reflect on whether I wanted to protest and if it would be the right decision.

Could I justify the risk, the potential repercussions, when life pulsed so preciously within me?

A stark realisation dawned on me that day: the only thing holding me back at this time was fear. I was wearing this suffocating cloak of society's expectations, stifling my potential. I realised that I had wasted years staying silent on many occasions when I could have used my voice. It was a heart-breaking truth; I had been playing a pale shadow of the vibrant, courageous person I could be.

My colleagues were mostly supportive, cheering me on during the media appearances I was now making, mainly on radio. They would eagerly share my articles and videos, but when the word 'protest' tumbled out of my mouth, their once enthusiastic cheer turned into silence.

While waiting for the results of my oral glucose tolerance test, I made a few phone calls to gauge how other doctors would feel if we went ahead with the decision to protest. Here are a few of the things that my colleagues told me that day. They linger in my memory, a constant reminder of the battle I fought within myself to take this brave step.

'Meenal, there is enough PPE. The government has put out urgent calls for companies to supply protective gear to hospitals. If you protest, you will look and sound stupid.'

'You're pregnant. You shouldn't be doing any of this; your family will get so upset seeing their pregnant daughter going out in public and having her face on TV.'

'If you protest, you will look like an extremist. I don't know why you feel the government isn't doing enough. You've got no chance against such a big establishment. It will crush you.'

> *'Is Nishant forcing you to do this? This doesn't sound like something you would do.'*

The last comment hit a nerve. I was very capable of making my own decisions and having my own thought processes. There seems to be a misunderstanding in our South Asian culture that the men usually make the major decisions and the women silently follow. Nishant had put his neck on the line just a few weeks ago and the story was all about him and his stance on the pandemic. Unfortunately, society expected me to sit silently behind him and watch.

Thankfully, I've been very fortunate to have found a life partner who believes in none of that. Nishant wanted to work with me; he wanted to hold my hand and fight this together. We each had strengths that we could use to our advantage and we functioned as a team, working towards one goal – justice.

After my first two phone calls, I realised how much energy I was pouring into justifying our decision to protest. It was draining me of any energy I had, which wasn't very much at this stage of my pregnancy. I could have been using that energy to think about ways to protest and help other people. These comments were hurtful, but I used that disappointment as fuel to show everyone that despite how helpless we were all feeling, change was possible.

I'd like to also point out that at this stage, I hadn't even mentioned this to my parents. They didn't even have a clue about what was going on in my head. All they knew was that a pregnant nurse had died and I was upset by it. I didn't know how to start explaining myself to them; it seemed like another battle which I just had no energy for.

As I drove home aftet my glucose test, the road unfurled

before me like a life path, dotted with crossroads of decisions. It was time to curate my own support system, not just cheerleaders, but wise counsel. I wasn't looking for blind praise; I needed a tribe to help me readjust my moral compass in moments of difficulty.

I can't remember a time where I was so focused on a goal. I seemed to have activated a hidden chamber in my brain; this was a side of me I never knew existed. By this point, this is all I was thinking about. Every second of my day was dedicated to planning my protest. But despite this focus, fear was a bitter pill I had to swallow, and feelings of uncertainty were part of the process. I was in a constant state of doubt. I had these questions echoing in my head day and night: What if nobody else took notice? What if nothing changes? How would my family react?

But sitting idly and being complicit felt like a slow, suffocating poison, a betrayal of everything Nishant and I believed in.

Nishant and I wanted to protest on the morning of Sunday 19 April as it would have marked one week after Nurse Mary's death. This meant that I had around 48 hours to plan it. But his trust, a silent language we'd honed over years, resonated between us. It was in his weary eyes, the unspoken plea, 'Make this right, make it count.' The weight of that trust settled on my shoulders, a comforting yet terrifying burden.

I arrived home from my glucose appointment and called Manjit. She had put her neck on the line several times throughout her career as an activist. She fought against cultural taboos and took many unconventional routes to raise awareness about periods through her charity. I knew she would get me in the right headspace.

We spoke at length about how I was feeling about everything. She knew I was upset and wanted to drive my emotions into something positive. Manjit very delicately and respectfully interrogated my thought process. She wanted to know why I felt this was so important and what outcome I wanted to achieve from it. There was never a point in this conversation where I felt intimidated or unheard; she was guiding me through my own thought process and giving me the clarity I needed. She emphasised that every action I took from here on would have a consequence. I just had to decide if those consequences were worth it and if I was mentally prepared to tackle them head on.

After speaking to Manjit, I remembered one of my old school teachers, Lizanne. Officially in school, she was Mrs Pardo but after I went to university, we stayed in touch and became very close friends. Our friendship blossomed throughout my time in medical school and our previous formal student-teacher relationship turned into a friendship where we would seek advice from each other and share our happiest and most challenging moments in our lives. Lizanne has two young girls, whom I've babysat and adore deeply. I wanted to know how she felt as a mother of two young girls. What would she do if she was in my position? How would she want her daughters to be inspired by their mother's behaviour and actions?

As expected, there was an element of worry when I spoke to Lizanne. Despite some of her doubts, she still encouraged me to continue with what I felt was right. The world was in a state of constant fear and worry. The media and the internet were causing so many of us around the world so much distress. We needed hope. The world needed the reassurance that despite so many odds stacked against us at the time, there were people still fighting to help ease the blow of all the deaths and suffering we were witnessing.

'Meenal, you need to portray yourself as a beacon of hope. I want people to see you protest and feel that you're standing by them. You're standing by every individual around the world watching you, hand by hand, helping them through this crisis.'

These are Lizanne's own words:

As the Covid-19 pandemic swept across the world, I watched in awe and fear as healthcare workers bravely faced the frontlines. Among them were my dear friends, Meenal and Nishant, both dedicated doctors working tirelessly in the emergency unit. My heart couldn't help but ache for them, especially Meenal, who was six months pregnant during this critical time.

I had known Meenal since she was a young child, and our bond has only grown stronger over the years (she's my little sister now). From being her table tennis coach to becoming her friend and GCSE teacher, I had seen her passion for helping others flourish. However, witnessing her now enduring the challenges of being a frontline healthcare worker while carrying her unborn child filled me with concern.

I tried my best to offer Meenal comfort and support, encouraging her to be cautious and prioritise her safety. The thought of my dear friend facing such dangers during her pregnancy was almost too much to bear.

When Mary Agyapong died from Covid-19 shortly after giving birth, the news hit Meenal hard, fuelling her determination to fight for justice for all healthcare workers facing similar risks. I could hear the pain in her voice during our conversations, but also heard her unyielding resolve to make a difference.

Refusing to be silenced, Meenal decided to take a stand and participate in a protest at Parliament. She wanted to shed light on the dire shortage of essential supplies and the media gagging faced by NHS staff. I was proud of her bravery, but my worry for her safety only grew as she ventured into the heart of the fight. She asked for my advice and support. I thought it was pointless to try and deter her; I knew her too well. So I supported her drive and vision. I knew she would be well cared for with Nishant by her side.

As she prepared her speech for the protest, I offered my support and lent an ear to her thoughts. We had long conversations about the risks she was taking, and I tried to provide encouragement and guidance in crafting her powerful words. I knew she had the strength and determination to make an impact, but her responsibility weighed heavily on her and it made me uncomfortable with worry too.

We spent time discussing the content and tone of her speech. I knew it was crucial to strike a balance between acknowledging the grim reality of the situation and inspiring hope for a better future. I wanted her words to resonate with the decision-makers and the public, urging them to take action and support the frontline heroes.

While her initial draft conveyed anger, desperation and sadness, I encouraged Meenal to channel her exceptional qualities into the speech. I reminded her of her kind and compassionate nature, the care and love she showed her patients, and her unwavering bravery in the face of adversity. I wanted her to showcase these aspects of herself in her speech, painting a picture of the passionate and dedicated healthcare worker she truly was.

We also discussed the importance of being constructive in her approach. Instead of merely highlighting the problems, I urged her to suggest solutions and a way forward. This would show that the healthcare workers were not just complaining, but actively seeking improvements and support. I told her to be a beacon of hope.

Meenal's speech needed to be a call for action and empathy. I encouraged her to appeal to the hearts of the listeners, asking them to imagine the challenges faced by frontline workers and the patients who relied on their care. This approach would foster a sense of unity and understanding, motivating others to stand alongside the healthcare workers in their fight for better protection and support. She took a big risk to represent not only herself but also countless other passionate and dedicated healthcare professionals who deserved to be heard. By uniting together, their voices would be stronger, and their message harder to ignore.

In the end, Meenal's speech transformed into a powerful and moving call to action. It eloquently expressed her anger and sadness at the challenging circumstances faced by NHS staff, but it also portrayed her as a strong, compassionate and resilient advocate for change.

Her words ignited a spark among the crowd, sparking a movement for positive change. The impact was profound, as her speech reached decision-makers and the public, drawing attention to the plight of healthcare workers and the urgent need for better protection and support.

As I watched her on the news, I felt a sense of pride and admiration for my brave friend. She had turned her

> *emotions and concerns into a powerful force for good, inspiring others to stand up and make a difference. Meenal's protest had become a powerful call for action, guided by empathy and hope.*

This is exactly what I needed.

While I did receive support from some colleagues during critical moments when I spoke up, the idea of protesting or taking a stand felt deeply unsafe and risky. Perhaps those around me who had been disappointed by my actions and disapproval saw me as simply being angry, not fully understanding the weight of the concerns I was trying to raise. Nobody wants to see an angry woman protesting on TV during a time of distress. I wanted to come across as someone who would stand boldly to protect my colleagues. I also wanted to send a clarion call to colleagues around the world and show them that if they're not happy with the state of affairs, they have a voice and the power to take action. There was just one thing that made me uncomfortable – the colour of my skin.

How would people react if they saw a South Asian pregnant woman on TV taking a stand against the British Establishment? Would it make people uncomfortable and subsequently open me up to more abuse?

If there was one excuse that I would find to talk myself out of this, it was this one. There was a chance my protest would be on the local news. At that time, I didn't expect it to go viral around the world and so I thought I'd be able to put a lid on things if I had to. Looking back, I was working under one mantra: 'Act now, deal with the consequences later.'

There was no time to ponder or worry. We had to get moving.

Chapter 7

THE PROTEST

Protests are a form of political expression that have been used throughout history to raise awareness of issues and to demand change. The first recorded protests in history took place in ancient Egypt. In 1878, archaeologists discovered a papyrus scroll that contained a record of a protest that took place in the city of Memphis in 1159 BC. The protest was organised by a group of farmers who were angry about the high taxes that they were being forced to pay. The farmers marched on the palace of the pharaoh and demanded that he lower their taxes. The pharaoh eventually agreed to lower the taxes, and the protest was successful.

Demanding better pay, protection and working conditions has been threaded into our society for centuries. Protests can take different forms and the most effective resonate with the public, allowing them to empathise with a cause. Striking has also been a popular form of protest. In 2015, junior doctors in England went on strike for the first time in 40 years, over a new contract that the government had proposed, which would have seen the doctors working longer hours and being paid less. The strike lasted for nine days, and had a significant impact on the NHS. It was estimated to have cost the NHS

£100 million due to cancelled appointments and increased overtime pay for non-striking NHS staff. The strike was a major event in the history of the NHS, and many people felt a sense of solidarity with junior doctors, who were seen as being unfairly treated by the government.

I felt that a one-woman protest could be effective because it would have been difficult for anyone in the press or in Parliament to ignore. They might be able to ignore numbers on a page, but a heavily pregnant woman standing in their shadow, a living embodiment of the consequences, that would be a story they wouldn't be able to spin.

There was a striking image I had come across in medical school one day as I was randomly scrolling on the internet. It came back to me as I was planning my protest. It was a vivid reminder of the power of a single voice, a single act.

The Tank Man photo, taken by Jeff Widener on 5 June 1989, is one of the most iconic images of the Tiananmen Square protests. The protests were sparked by the death of Hu Yaobang, a former Communist Party leader who had been known for his liberal policies. The protests quickly grew to include a wide range of demands, including greater democracy, freedom of speech and an end to corruption.

The photo shows a lone man standing in front of a column of tanks that were moving into Tiananmen Square to disperse the protesters. The man, who has never been identified, refused to move even as the tanks tried to pass him. The photo was widely circulated around the world and became a symbol of the Chinese people's resistance to government oppression.

The Tank Man photo went viral for several reasons. First, it was a powerful image that captured the attention of people around the world. The man's defiance in the face of overwhelming odds was inspiring and resonated with people who were fighting for their own freedom. Second, the photo was widely circulated by the media. Newspapers, magazines and television stations around the world ran the photo, which helped to spread the story of the Tiananmen Square protests. In the years since the photo was taken, social media has become a powerful tool for spreading information and images. The Tank Man photo has been shared millions of times on social media, which has helped to keep the story of the Tiananmen Square protests alive.

The Tank Man photo had a significant impact on creating change. It offered a powerful and undeniable image of the situation. The Tiananmen Square protests were under tight media control, making the photo a rare glimpse of the event. The photo also inspired people around the world to fight for their own freedom. In the years since the photo was taken, there have been many protests and demonstrations inspired by the Tank Man. The photo has also been used as a symbol of hope and resistance by people who are fighting for freedom and democracy.

The Tank Man photo is a powerful reminder of the power of one person to stand up to oppression. It is a symbol of hope and resistance that continues to inspire people around the world. This is an example of a protest which is unarguably powerful and effective.

There have been instances where protests have been controversial because of the tactics that are used by protesters, which can be seen as disruptive or even violent, such as blocking traffic or vandalising property. These tactics can alienate people who might otherwise support the cause of the protest, and they can also lead to arrests and prosecutions. The media coverage of protests can also influence how controversial they are. If the media focuses on the negative aspects of protests, such as violence or disruption, this can make them more controversial.

Just Stop Oil* is a climate change activist group that was founded in the UK in October 2021. The group's stated goal is to 'bring about a just transition to a fossil fuel free future'. Just Stop Oil has been criticised for its use of disruptive protests, such as blocking roads in London and glueing themselves to the entrance of the Shell headquarters. In November 2021, group members glued themselves to the pitch at an English Premier League football match.

There are a number of reasons why people disagree with Just Stop Oil's forms of protests. Some people believe that the protests are disruptive and inconvenience the public. Others disagree with the group's goals, arguing that they are too radical or that they will not be effective in addressing climate change.

Just Stop Oil is a controversial group, but it is clear that they are passionate about their cause. The group's protests have raised awareness of the climate crisis, and they have put pressure on the government to take action. Whether or not the protests are effective, they are certainly having a big impact.

The right to protest is protected by domestic legislation and the European Convention on Human Rights. However, the Conservative government made a number of changes to the law making it more difficult for people to exercise this right.

* https://juststopoil.org

Protests were illegal in the UK during April 2020, under the Coronavirus Act 2020. Section 63 of the Act prohibited 'gatherings on public land of more than two people'. This meant that any protest with more than two people was illegal, regardless of whether it was peaceful or not. There weren't any official rules for a one-woman protest and so I hoped that maybe, just maybe, I could get away with it.

* * *

An article in *The Guardian*, published in April 2020, stated:

> *At least 100 health and care workers have died of coronavirus, a nursing website has said, amid growing concerns about a lack of personal protective equipment (PPE) for those working on the frontline during the coronavirus pandemic.*[1]

The headlines were displaying statistics such as this on a daily basis, revealing that the supply of PPE was shambolic.

By this point, I had made it very clear to my senior colleagues and consultants that I was not going to accept working in a ward where the virus was present. I was happy to sit in an office and do hours and hours of admin if it meant staying away from the infected wards. One of my consultants was very supportive of my situation and allowed me to stay in one of the offices at the back of the hospital and work on discharge letters from patients who had previously left the hospital but had some paperwork to complete.

I was relatively safe at work, but I was still in the hospital watching porters push trolleys with body bags into the crematorium. I was witnessing families walk in and out of the hospital in tears, unable to console each other through their masks as they learned of the death of their loved ones. I was surrounded by so much grief and pain – it was palpable anywhere in the hospital. There was no escaping it.

By Friday, five days after Mary's passing, I had made my decision. I told my parents that I was going out to protest. I made it very clear that they weren't allowed to question my decision. It was as simple as that – nothing was up for debate any more. My usual warmth was replaced by an unfamiliar ruthlessness.

I had channelled my fear into something much more powerful – taking action.

I phoned Manjit that morning and asked her if she had any idea of how I could hold a sign up. Keep in mind, this was the first time I'd ever protested in my life. I had attended mass gatherings before, but I would blend into the crowd as a silent observer. I'd never physically made a placard, nor did I have a clue where to get placard-making equipment from. Manjit suggested ordering big white cards on Amazon, along with some marker pens, and said she would bring me some bamboo sticks to tape onto the back of the card for me to hold the sign.

Manjit travelled over 30 kilometres that morning to leave me some bamboo sticks. I had to attend a midwife appointment so I wasn't at home to see her, but she left a small note along with the sticks: 'Meenal, you've got this. We're all behind you.'

Some of my colleagues and family members were passionately against the idea of protesting at that time. I can count on just one hand the number of people who believed in my vision

– but that was enough. Relationships, for the moment, became a secondary concern. This cause, this fight, demanded my all, and I was prepared to give it, no matter the cost.

Nishant had spent the week dealing with Mary's husband, Ernest. Of course, we wanted to give him space, but we also wanted to ease the burden of the daily tasks he had at hand. Ernest had a huge responsibility; a newborn baby and a toddler who needed attention and activities to keep him busy. Nishant checked in on Ernest through Mary's colleagues who were also nurses and healthcare assistants in the hospital. Through them, we had an idea of what he needed to keep him going. As we were also preparing to welcome our own baby, I had a cupboard full of new clothes and gifts from relatives and friends. I decided to split it half and half between baby Mary and my own daughter.

As courtesy, Nishant had messaged Ernest to inform him of my protest and explain why I felt the need to go out and do this. Neither of us remembers the exact details of the conversation but I did know that Ernest was proudly supporting us. His grief was still fresh and at this point, I still don't think he had processed what had happened.

By Friday evening, I was writing down all the possible things I could write on my placard in my notebook.

- 'Protect doctors'
- 'Protect doctors with more PPE'
- 'Doctors are dying. We demand more PPE'
- 'NHS workers are suffering. Hold them to account'

I went through this list over and over again, trying to see which would have the most impact. I then realised that it wasn't just doctors who were suffering; it was nurses, healthcare assistants, ward clerks, cleaners and porters. I had to make a statement that embodied all staff. I spent hours thinking of a a phrase that was just three or four words to catch the eye of passersby or potential journalists. After a lot of consideration, I went with PROTECT HEALTHCARE WORKERS.

I got my pen and started drawing on my white canvas. My hands were shaking as I was writing the outline of these letters and it almost felt as if my hand was disconnected from my brain. My brain kept telling me that I should stop and nobody would even take notice of me holding the sign. But despite my brain creating these scenarios of failure, my hand just kept going. I kept on writing on my placard and colouring in the outlines as if I'd done this a million times before.

As I was working my way through my sign, Nishant walked back in from his shift.

'Meenal, we can't do this. I'm worried that we'll get in too much trouble. I feel as if they are following my movements.'

I couldn't believe what I was hearing. I had spent all week building myself up for this moment; I had had arguments with my own friends, I almost told my parents to stay out of my business and now Nishant, the person I needed the most, was waving a giant red danger flag.

I felt my heart sink for a moment. But this is how every doctor in the country was feeling. No doctor wanted to risk losing their medical licence or throwing their career away.

If every doctor conformed to the system, then nobody would ever protest. Nobody would ever speak up and history would never be able to document the real trauma and suffering that doctors were put through due to the negligence of the government. Nishant, who had his moment of courage and bravery after speaking to Carole, was almost a victim of the system – the system controlling the narrative of the pandemic across the country.

'Nishant, this is not okay. I refuse to just sit here and watch families be torn apart. Have you forgotten that baby Mary will never see her mother?' Tears were rolling down my cheeks as I was trying to explain why this had to be done.

'Meenal, I was called into one of my consultant's offices. I recently posted a short video on Twitter where I brought some donated hot food for a colleague who was sick with Covid-19 and they weren't happy with it.'

'Yes, and they won't be happy with anything you do.'

'But Meenal, they're telling me that I'm scare-mongering and they seem very unhappy with me. I cannot afford to lose anything right now. I just need to put my head down and get on with it.'

'You do, but I don't.'

Nobody knew me well enough at the time. Sure, I'd ruffled a few feathers previously for speaking to the media. But losing something? It never crossed my mind. Unlike my husband, who was stuck in the hamster wheel of speciality training, I had no strings attached. My focus was laser-sharp on the protest, a tunnel vision that blocked out potential repercussions. Reflecting back, it's clear I was swimming in a sea of naivety.

The sheer scale of the system I was poking with a stick?

Ignorant bliss.

Fear?

It simply wasn't in my vocabulary.

I was so invested in making this protest happen, I didn't even think of the consequences that could have been heading my way. My ignorance, a double-edged sword, had gifted me a fearless heart, but robbed me of foresight. On reflection, knowing what I know today, I'm not sure I'd feel as brave to go out and do what I did.

'Meenal, you're going to have to be the face of the protest then. I cannot be seen or heard or be anywhere near you.'

'That's fine, not a problem. Let's crack on.'

'Meenal, are you sure you'll be okay? You're pregnant. I don't want you to be worried or stressed. This could come with a whole other burden. You'll be rammed by the media; you'll be getting phone calls from your bosses. Are you sure you're ready for this?'

'Ernest is dealing with two children under the age of two. He's lost his wife. He's alone with no family in this country. Whatever I have to deal with is really a speck of dust in comparison.'

Nishant couldn't recognise me. The girl he knew, the one who always sat tucked into corners, who spoke in whispers, was gone. In her place stood a beacon of determination, her eyes blazing with a fire he'd never witnessed in the eight years that he'd known me.

My body language and my energy instilled a sense of faith and trust in Nishant. Considering all the difficult conversations he had to have over the last few weeks with his bosses, he knew I'd be able to handle anything coming my way.

We had our dinner, which by this point, was always just a simple spaghetti dish or I'd just dump vegetables in the oven. Healthcare worker perks gave us priority access to supermarkets, but access did little good when time itself was a scarce resource. Exhausted from 13-hour shifts, we found that elaborate meals were a distant memory. My mother had last visited just a few months earlier and filled our freezer with our favourite Indian dishes. At the time, when my mum was up until 1am preparing all the food for us before she left, it seemed as if we would never get through all of the food in time for her next visit. Who would have known that it would take a global pandemic to finish all the food my mum had prepared for us!

Through sheer tiredness and exhaustion, we managed to fall asleep. Just 24 hours stood between us and a decision that could alter the very fabric of our lives.

That Saturday, I spent my time upstairs alone in our guest room. I needed the silence, a vacuum to distil the chaos swirling around me. What would I say? Nishant and I existed in separate worlds that day, each of us focused on the execution and possible consequences of our decision.

I had a lot of details to think through. I couldn't allow anybody to make a single negative comment about my protest. A single misstep or a loose thread could have become the narrative. This protest, this fight for justice for Mary and countless grieving families, couldn't be hijacked by any stray comments. The weight of the message pressed down heavily, a responsibility that demanded every ounce of my focus. There was no room for error, not when the stakes were so high.

I had decided to wear scrubs as a sign to show that I was a healthcare worker. I also had to wear a mask – this may seem like a small part of the bigger picture, but this was one of the most important points I had to think about. I was protesting for better PPE, yet potentially using it for a purpose some would deem frivolous. In the end, I wore a reusable mask made by the lovely ladies at Binti International and I was hoping that for some time, people wouldn't be able to recognise me under the mask. Even if it bought me a few days of avoiding any confrontation with my bosses, it was enough.

With my stomach churning on nervous energy, I laid out my scrubs for the next morning on the sofa and went to sleep.

I woke up with the feeling of the sun rays hitting my skin that morning. I opened my eyes, turned to Nishant and whispered, 'Let's do this.'

I could feel the adrenaline running through me. It was the same feeling I had before sitting an exam or taking part in one of my competitive table tennis matches – I wanted to come out the other side winning. I left myself with no other option. And I believed I could win. I had spent the last week breathing every second and every moment of this protest.

I turned on the shower and as the water warmed up, I recited all the lines that I had prepared for the media that day. It was a pre-protest cram session, just like cramming for medical school finals, only this time the notes were seared into my memory with a fiercer urgency. I pictured my lines in my notebook; I emphasised the words that I had underlined and capitalised to explain the gravity of the situation. As I was going through my lines, I could feel Radhika kick inside me reminding me of my purpose – we were fighting for justice.

As I was getting out of the shower, Nishant knocked on the bathroom door and whispered, 'Don't forget my phone number.'

It took me a few seconds to make out what he meant. Nishant and I had spent the night before going through different scenarios which could get me in trouble. There were some stories going around the internet at that time of police stopping drivers on their commutes confirming where they were going and why they had left their house during lockdown.

We weren't afraid of questions. Our story, woven from the threads of truth – a late shift, a swollen belly, a concerned husband – was a shield against suspicion. We weren't worried about justifying our drive to London, but we were worried about me getting arrested.

Nishant grew up around central London and he knew most corners of the streets. He pointed out the choke points – the streets with a higher density of patrolling police and potential bottlenecks. It allowed us to visualise where exactly we might get stopped and where we would find each other if I had to make an exit. We had studied the roads and the area around Whitehall on Google Maps the night before using Google Street View. Nishant had pointed out where he would park the car, drop me off and then meet me a couple of hours later. I knew exactly how many metres I had to walk from my drop-off point to Number 10 and how long that walk would take me. It meant that if I wasn't at a certain point at a certain time, Nishant could prepare for any trouble coming our way. My protest became a choreographed act of defiance.

Nishant reminded me that morning that I had to write his phone number on the inside of my bicep, under my sleeve in case I had to contact him for any emergency. I quickly got changed, wrote Nishant's number with a marker, grabbed a packet of biscuits from the kitchen and waited in the car. I was almost reciting my lines by this point like a mantra. As I was whispering them to myself in the car, Nishant popped around the corner and joked, 'You haven't forgotten your sign, have you?'

I'd put my placard in the back of the car the night before, along with my work identity badge to show police officers that I was commuting from work. This operation had to be executed perfectly – my life and the lives of so many other healthcare workers depended on it. I couldn't risk leaving anything behind.

Nishant started the engine and as he turned the key, he asked me one more time, 'Are you sure you want to do this? Remember, you don't have to do anything that makes you uncomfortable.'

'Nishant, just drive please. Don't waste time.'

He didn't respond, but from the nod of his head, I could tell he knew that I wasn't turning back at this point.

As we drove down the motorway, the silence was a stark reminder of how the world around us had completely changed. From busy commuters and noisy engines occupying the motorways, to empty roads and complete silence. Nishant and I didn't say a single word to each other the whole way. Physically, we were in the car, but mentally, we were both running through the execution of my protest. When we arrived at our parking spot, I walked towards the boot of the car, took my sign and nodded at Nishant.

We walked in opposite directions.

The next time we would make eye contact would be when I was standing outside Number 10.

* * *

As I walked down Whitehall and looked up at the buildings around me, I realised how trapped I was within the hospital. There was a huge contrast between the reality I was living and what I was walking through that Sunday morning.

Spring was in full bloom and nature was bringing a lot of colour into our very difficult lives during the pandemic. But the only colours my eyes were accustomed to at the time were colours of danger and flashing lights. I had forgotten how it felt to look at a pink flower blossoming from its bud on a tree and how beautiful it was to watch the sun's rays fall through the leaves of the tall trees around me.

I had to stop myself in my train of thought as I started to drift off into a different world – a world where the virus didn't exist and people were enjoying the beauty nature had to offer. As I continued walking down Whitehall, I watched cyclists ride past, members of the public carrying out their daily exercise, and I paid attention to the posters stuck on the lampposts as I made my way towards Number 10.

Usually, I would walk straight past posters around Whitehall as there is so much going on around this area. Many people protest on various subjects and it can be quite jarring to walk past so many people screaming down megaphones about political and social issues they're passionate about. That Sunday morning was different, however. I felt as if I was in a vacuum. The roads were empty and the silence gave me some space to fully absorb what was around me.

Some posters were messages to NHS staff and essential workers to say thank you and expressed how much the British public appreciated their efforts. These posters made me smile. For the first time, I felt that people genuinely cared.

There were other posters, however, which struck me. They were neon green and although they were small and A4 sized, you could spot them from a mile away due to their brightly coloured nature.

'Thank you, Boris' was the headline of these posters.

I refused to read the rest because it felt as if the whole of Whitehall and Downing Street was living in their own bubble of self-created propaganda which completely distanced them from frontline workers like myself. I smiled under my mask because I knew that people would read these neon-coloured posters and then see my sign, which sent out completely the opposite message. The contrast was stark but perhaps very much needed to remind me and others who walked past me that day of how NHS workers were living completely different realities to our politicians.

After about ten minutes, I reached my spot. I was outside the gates at Number 10 and although I had an idea of where Nishant could be, I couldn't see him. I knew he'd taken a different route which would take slightly longer, but not seeing him around made me nervous. I had policemen behind me guarding the gates; my hands were sweaty and I couldn't get myself to hold my sign up. I froze for a few seconds and was about to turn around and walk back. All of a sudden, all of that bravery and fierce courage I had shown to Nishant over the last few days had melted away.

But then I felt a kick in my womb.

Radhika jolted me out of this paralysing fear and I remembered why I had made this decision in the first place – to seek justice for Nurse Mary's family.

At this point, I caught Nishant's eye as he was on the road opposite me. Behind him, I could see the London Eye, which was now empty and completely stationary. As I lifted my sign, I felt my shoulders stand taller and my spine straighten. My confidence was coming back to me as I lifted my chin up and stood firmly outside the gates of Downing Street with my placard.

My memories of that hour: pin drop silence, cyclists riding past giving me a wave of solidarity and gentle movements from Radhika as she kicked in my womb. My unborn child was a poignant reminder of my true purpose. I had reporters walk past me as I had expected and I was photographed and interviewed – none of this fazed me. I recited my rehearsed lines loud and proud as they questioned why I felt the need to protest. As I stood outside for over an hour, I felt a tingling feeling in my ankles – a symptom of prolonged standing during pregnancy. I also started to feel a bit nauseous because I hadn't eaten much that morning and was running purely on adrenaline.

After I'd stood outside for over two hours, Nishant signalled from the other side of the road and I walked across to him. He asked me if I was okay and gave me some water to drink.

'I think we've done our job. Let's hope something comes out of this.' I was getting breathless and the exhaustion was starting to hit me as the adrenaline was wearing off.

Nishant grabbed my sign, held my hand tightly and told me how proud he was of me.

We walked back to the car, oblivious to what was going to hit us next.

* * *

I'd done it! As a South Asian, pregnant doctor, I stood outside the gates of Downing Street and protested for the rights of my colleagues during a global pandemic. I walked away with Nishant with my head held high and a spring in my step. I knew that this was just the beginning.

I had so much more I wanted to give to this fight; I had so much more to give to the families who were fighting for justice.

Finally, I felt that I truly believed in everything I was doing. I wasn't pretending to be brave any more; I wasn't pretending to be someone I wasn't. That one protest put all the unknown pieces together. These were the pieces of the jigsaw where I questioned my values and beliefs and tried to deduce the kind of feminist and mother I wanted to be for my daughter. I didn't want to be too loud, too angry or too aggressive. But I also didn't want to be too soft or meek. I kept searching for inspiration around me to mirror the behaviours of other activists and change-makers I personally looked up to. I wish I'd known that I'd had it within me the whole time, and that I didn't have to look outside myself. It was within me the whole time.

That's the beauty of activism which seems to be missed – we are all activists in our own unique sense and it's our individual ways of expressing our beliefs which allows society to change in so many ways.

Nishant asked me how I was feeling and all I could say was, 'I feel bloody great!'

It was as if I had passed an exam at medical school; all the weight was off my shoulders. I could go to sleep at night knowing that despite the unjust treatment of so many families and the lack of accountability and consequences that our politicians were facing, I had done my very best and hadn't simply accepted that the world around me should continue as it was.

We walked back to our car and made our way home. As soon as I sat down, the exhaustion hit me. The days leading up to the protest were very intense. I was battling so many emotions. I was dealing with the opinions of my loved ones and my close friends and trying to juggle all of that and come to my own conclusions. My head felt heavy, my legs felt weak and I was definitely very dehydrated. As soon as we got home, I took a cold shower, lay down on the sofa and gulped a cold glass of water. Before I knew it, I'd fallen asleep. I had no idea what I was about to wake up to.

There was one Meenal who existed before the protest, and there is the Meenal of today. The Meenal who existed before the protest had no idea of the endless possibilities that could exist purely through sheer determination and self-belief. I woke up from that nap feeling like a new woman.

I was writing a new chapter of my life now. The new Meenal was ready to take on the world.

I had slept for a good four or five hours. My protest photos and interviews from that morning had enough time to circulate the internet by this point. In fact, it really doesn't take more than a few minutes for something to go viral online these days. Imagine what a few hours had done!

Nishant had messaged Carole Cadwalladr to tell her about my protest. She replied saying, 'Meenal is my hero!'

I thought to myself, 'Wow, Carole knows about my protest. How cool is that?'

She was just one person, but how do you react when over 4000 people are praising your actions online? There is no way to process so much information and react and thank every individual. Our brains cannot process so much in such a short time. At the same time, I had the same relatives and friends who were against everything I did, messaging me and telling me how brave I was.

So, there I was, in my living room, with my phone in my hand, wondering why so many strangers were showing their solidarity. It baffled me that I had doctors dotted across the world showing their support, yet my own close friends and family, who I'd known for years, had rejected the idea of a protest.

My Twitter following shot up from 20 followers to over 2000 that night. That one photo, which was taken so perfectly, caught the very essence of what the protest was all about: a determined pregnant doctor standing up for her fellow doctors and nurses. This photo was taken by Associated Press (AP), which meant that any story they had written on me would be distributed to media channels across the world.

Nishant was right. This protest would change my life forever.

Chapter 8

UNMASKING THE TRUTH

Our Legal Battle for Justice

April 2020: The defiant echoes of my solo protest outside Downing Street still hung in the air. One week after my protest, Nishant received a message on Twitter. It was from a retired GP, a veteran of the medical field who had been stirred by Nishant's words in *The Guardian*. Impressed by his courage, he floated a daring idea, a legal challenge – to hold the government's feet to the fire, to force it to answer for its mishandling of the pandemic.

In our work, we were exposed to high viral loads of coronavirus over a prolonged period of time so we needed the highest protection from infection. The government claimed to be guided by science. It was clear that its failure to supply the right PPE in sufficient amounts was making it adjust the guidelines on the use of PPE that do not meet World Health Organization or Health and Safety standards.

Nishant, initially cautious, felt a spark ignite after a few phone calls. The legal route felt like a scalpel, a precise weapon to dissect the government's failings. We were still reeling from Mary's loss, raw and desperate for answers. The fight, daunting as it was, felt like a necessary extension of our grief, even if it piled on to our overflowing plates.

We knew that the legal costs would be extortionate and we were in no position to pay any of this by ourselves, so we discussed using a crowdfunder to help us raise money to pay our lawyer and fund for the case. We had to raise over £80,000 to cover all our lawyer's costs, our meetings and all the admin that came along with this legal battle. But for us, the fight for justice was non-negotiable. This time, the target wasn't the virus itself, but the system that failed to protect those on the frontlines.

The fight was far from easy. The government's slow response added to the frustration. Our perseverance was fuelled by a deep sense of responsibility for our colleagues and a growing public outcry. Our story resonated with the public, garnering media attention and support from fellow doctors.

It was wonderful we were all clapping on Thursday evenings, but it was also critical that frontline NHS staff had the proper masks, visors, gowns, gloves and so on, so that we could get on and help patients without fear of catching the virus ourselves and spreading it further.

We were challenging the government guidance on the basis that:

- PPE guidelines were not in line with the international standards set by the World Health Organization or domestic legislation regarding health and safety at work
- it exposed healthcare workers to greater risks of contracting Covid-19 and failed to address the greater risks faced by BAME healthcare workers

- it was unclear and had resulted in inconsistent practices across NHS Trusts
- it failed to make clear the level of risk faced by healthcare workers depending on the level of PPE they could access, or that healthcare workers had a right to refuse to work without adequate PPE
- it fell short of recommendations previously published by Public Health England.

We were also asking for the government to consider the particular risk that BAME healthcare workers faced with coronavirus and the higher proportion of deaths among healthcare workers.

Flipping through the diary entries and Crowdjustice fundraising page from our legal battle feels like reliving a tidal wave. Not a wave of fear or uncertainty, but a wave of gratitude that still washes over me. The outpouring of messages and donations from the public was breathtaking. It was a stark reminder that the NHS wasn't just our institution; it was theirs. This wasn't just our fight; it was their fight for the healthcare system they cherished. Witnessing that support, that willingness to chip in, was emotionally overwhelming in the best way possible.

Here are some excerpts from the crowdfunding diary and letters to our supporters.

27 APRIL 2020: FROM THE CROWDFUNDING DIARY

Initially, we need to raise £60,000 for our legal costs, including representation and barristers, adverse cost protection and court fees, so that we can take action as quickly as possible if the government does not revise the guidance and take adequate steps to source PPE to prevent the unnecessary loss of life among health workers. We will then need to move quickly to a larger stretch target of £120,000, so that we can pursue the action to a full hearing if necessary.

The government has delayed its response to our crucial PPE challenge, while doctors and healthcare professionals continue to be exposed to Covid-19.

Thanks so much for your support. We wanted to give an update on the government response to our claim and provide more detailed information about why this case is so critically important.

Our lawyers have heard back from the government. Despite the serious issues raised by our claim, as confirmed in the BBC *Panorama* report broadcast yesterday evening, the Government Legal Department (representing the Secretary of State and Public Health England) has said they will get back to us by the end of the week. In the meantime, the guidance on PPE, and efforts to source PPE, remain inadequate, putting the lives of healthcare workers, their families and ultimately their patients at greater risk than needs to be the case. Our lawyers have asked for a response by Wednesday afternoon, in light of this urgency.

Thanks to your support, our case has already made international headlines in *The Guardian*[1] and on Reuters.[2] Help us to continue to push the government to ensure healthcare workers are properly protected by adequate PPE and have the right to refuse to work when they do not.

This challenge is about protecting *all* NHS workers on the frontline.

We believe that the government is failing to protect front-line NHS workers[3] because of a lack of adequate PPE.

This is because:

- UK PPE guidance[4] falls short of standards set by the WHO
- the government has not taken adequate steps to address the PPE shortage.

Tragically, over 100 healthcare workers have already died[5] from coronavirus, and countless more are infected. This has disproportionately affected workers of a BAME background.

This is a breach of the government's international obligation to protect the lives of healthcare workers under Article 2 of the European Convention on Human Rights, and a breach of the Health and Safety at Work Act 1974.

We want the government to act now to remedy the current shortages in PPE, and to clarify its guidance.

What have we done so far?

Our lawyers at Bindmans have sent a pre-action letter inviting the government to:

- review current PPE guidance and bring it in line with WHO standards
- confirm that urgent steps have been taken to engage with the European Union's PPE bulk buying programme[6]
- investigate the deaths of healthcare workers, in particular why BAME healthcare workers are disproportionately affected.

They have also requested disclosure of the research and evidence base which informed changes to the PPE guidance on 17 April, particularly because the Royal Colleges were not consulted[7] before these amendments were introduced.

We had sought a reply by 4pm on Monday 27 April, but the Secretary of State and Public Health England's lawyers have asked for an additional five days to provide a response. Given the urgency, our lawyers have asked for a reply by Wednesday.

1 MAY 2020: LETTER TO OUR SUPPORTERS

In true doctor style, we ask you to please take a seat – we've got some good news and some bad news...

The good news

- Our solicitors are doing a fantastic job, and we've received plenty of public support. We have pressed the government to respond, regularly. Our team is superb, and we have some creative surprises on the way.
- Meenal featured on *Good Morning Britain* opposite Matt Hancock, where he admitted for the first time that PPE guidelines were based on supply, not science. This makes it very clear that the government has knowingly sent healthcare workers into dangerous situations. Headlines have unfortunately been off the mark, so to make absolutely clear: *we are not suing the government.* We have merely asked Matt Hancock a simple question: *Where is your evidence?*

- The *Daily Mail* has endorsed our campaign, and featured a full-page op-ed from Meenal on Thursday. She emphasised that if we have British manufacturers at our disposal, why are we flying in supplies from Burma?[8]

The bad news

- We are deeply disappointed by the government's failure to respond to us in a prompt manner. Doctors and nurses are falling ill every day, and we have only asked them simple questions. Our legal team are frustrated by this, and we feel we now have to take charge and say: *This is not good enough.*
- In other bad news, Meenal is feeling the baby kick very hard indeed. We suspect it is out of dissatisfaction at Matt Hancock's persistent inaccuracies over PPE, testing, and the like.

What next?

We need to act fast. We need to reach our initial target of £60,000 within 21 days, and our stretch target of £120,000 will see us through a judicial review.

Thank you for already contributing – we still need your help.

If you can please share with your friends via WhatsApp, Twitter and Facebook – this will be the most effective way of spreading our message and ensuring that we meet our target.

Unlike Matt Hancock, let's try reaching our target without moving the numbers...

3 MAY 2020: FROM THE CROWDFUNDING DIARY

Still no answer.

Excellent news – thanks to a stunning grassroots response, we have raised over £10,000 in the space of just a few days!

Regrettably, Matt Hancock has spent the last few days boasting about dubious testing targets instead of answering our legal team's email.

Keep in mind, we have only asked for simple evidence from the government, which should be freely and easily available. Hell, at this stage, we'd even accept a link to a Wikipedia page that shows us why it's acceptable for our colleagues to work on the frontline with a dinner lady's apron.

It's dead simple: just show us the evidence, and we will have no need to pursue this further.

Meenal would like to add that she ideally wants to deliver the baby in hospital, and not in the High Court. This is on you, Matt.

7 MAY 2020: LETTER TO OUR SUPPORTERS

Will there be no end to the scandals?

> *There are perfectly adequate stocks of PPE in this country... PPE issues have been completely resolved. (Dr Jenny Harries, 20 March 2020)*[9]

We didn't believe it back then. We definitely don't believe it now. Forty-eight per cent of the national stockpile was *out of date*, and our Deputy Chief Medical Officer had the audacity to say that we need 'more adult conversation' about PPE.

This is disgraceful. Shameful.

The government will never admit to its faults and will not come clean about its egregious errors.

We have still not heard back from Matt Hancock's team – two weeks on, they keep asking for more time. It's already too late.

We need to seek justice via a judicial review.

Our government does not value the lives of doctors and nurses. We must hold it accountable, and make sure one thing is clear: never again.

Wash your hands,
Dr Meenal Viz and Dr Nishant Joshi

12 MAY 2020: LETTER TO OUR SUPPORTERS

Finally, an answer!

Good things often come to those who wait...this is not one of those times. We are grateful for having received a response from Matt Hancock's legal team. But, after discussing the government's reply with our expert team of lawyers, we have asked for a few further clarifications.

To summarise, our challenge centres around a simple question: *Has the British government sent doctors and nurses to work in environments without providing appropriate PPE?*

In the spirit of transparency, openness and honesty, we have asked the government if it would allow for publication of its reply to us. We believe that government decisions should be open to scrutiny, and that its decision-making processes deserve closer inspection.

To be clear, we want to help the government arrive at the best decisions – Meenal's tummy is growing to the point where she feels 'like a balloon about to pop' (her own words), and so if we were spared the thought of delivering our baby in the High Court in July, we'd be ever so grateful.

In the first instance, a Zoom call where we could put our points across would be massively helpful.

We will update as soon as we hear from Mr Hancock's team again.

In the meantime, please do keep sharing our link on Facebook groups and pages. We really need your help to see this through.

PS: Meenal has intimated that if you help us reach our stretch target by donating the most funds, she will allow you to choose the baby's name. So long as it's not Priti.

13 MAY 2020: LETTER TO OUR SUPPORTERS

You wanted to see the government's response. It has refused.

Matt Hancock does not want you to see his reply to us. What is he hiding?

We requested full transparency throughout these hearings – and we insist that all correspondence between our team and Matt Hancock needs to be fully public. He has declined to do so.

It is a matter of national interest and it does not sit right with us that in a case that centres around transparency, he does not want to be fully transparent.

Oh boy.

* * *

To date, we have taken things logically and calmly. We initially raised local concerns, and then realised these issues were of a time-critical nature and so Nishant became the first frontline doctor to speak publicly[10] about the impending PPE crisis.

After the tragic passing of our dear pregnant nurse Mary Agyapong,[11] we decided that enough was enough. Meenal – then six months pregnant – took the brave step of protesting outside Downing Street with her now iconic sign.

We initially attempted to engage the government through formal channels, using a legal route that required an official government response.[12] While we did eventually receive a response from their legal team two months after our initial letter, the government's engagement was insufficient, and they continue to obstruct our pursuit of justice.

This should have never happened – but with your help we can ensure that this never happens again.

Please keep sharing our link with your friends, family and rich uncles who believe that justice needs to be served.

Best regards,
Dr Nishant Joshi & Dr Meenal Viz
(Our 31 week foetus sends its warmest regards)

24 MAY 2020: LETTER TO OUR SUPPORTERS

We appreciate that you have been in touch with our lawyers over the past few weeks. But our communications have exclusively been via our own lawyers, and obviously things have become a bit tetchy so we just wanted to reset proceedings and reintroduce ourselves.

We don't want to be doing this. We didn't plan on doing this. We're doctors in a pandemic. We want to focus on saving lives and stitching this country back together. Frankly, in our limited time off, we would both rather be phoning our families and getting our baby's cot together. We haven't seen our families in nearly three months.

But we have been pushed into taking action.

All we want is to sit in our small garden, enjoy the sunshine and watch the grass grow long while we sip on tea and eat scones.

We acknowledge and respect that you prefer for your correspondence to remain private, and we will respect this – I hope that a public acknowledgement of your preference is not in itself considered to be an egregious breach of confidence. But nevertheless, in the interests of full transparency, we feel it is important to publicly acknowledge your private desire to not make public your communications for the time being.

Anyway, we digress.

Reading between the lines, we know that you frequent this Crowdjustice page very often, and so this is a simple Bank Holiday assurance from us – we want to make your life easier.

If you are willing to release emails, disclose documents, and engage in healthy and constructive dialogue that addresses our ongoing serious concerns, we would be most obliged.

Also, we note your repeated emails making clear that you are operating under significant operational pressures... It is now midnight on Sunday night, and Nishant has completed a 65-hour week taking care of sick children. Meanwhile, we have fielded further phone calls from families of bereaved healthcare workers.

It is our duty and obligation to do our best for these good people, and to avoid similar citizens suffering the same fate in the weeks, months and years to come.

We need answers from Matt Hancock and we are willing to work with your department in order to achieve practicable solutions. That can only come with an initial acknowledgement and apology. As doctors, we have a duty of candour to our patients – if things go wrong, we have to 'fess up' and say that things could have been done better.

Nobody expected this pandemic to run smoothly – least of all doctors! But there have been obvious and egregious PPE failures that need to be addressed.

Thank you for your continued willingness to engage with us so that we can protect healthcare workers.

12 JULY 2020: LETTER TO OUR SUPPORTERS

We have filed for judicial review.

That's it. That's the update.

We have been deeply unhappy with the government's replies to our pleas for help. We have garnered mainstream media attention in broadsheet papers,[13] our protests have gained support from doctors,[14] while our article on systemic racism[15] went viral, and was discussed by senior members of PHE and NHS England, and by members of Parliament.

Importantly, our campaigning has become part of public consciousness. From a 'niche' issue of PPE, we have been able to put pressure on other important issues, such as rights for pregnant workers and rights for BAME healthcare workers.

We appreciate that you have given us a platform to speak up, and with that comes a responsibility to be ambassadors for truth, honesty and integrity.

As doctors, our fundamentals are clear: we want to lessen suffering. Many families have continued to get in touch with us, explaining how they have suffered at the hands of systematic failings.

To these families, we will make one commitment: we will seek justice for you.

Thank you for your help and support so far – we now have three major bodies on board with us as 'interested parties', showing the importance and far-reaching nature of our case.

PREGNANCY UPDATE: Meenal has now given birth to a beautiful baby girl (Radhika, meaning 'seeker of justice' in Sanskrit), and although we hit some health speedbumps (gestational diabetes is a real thing, so please attend your regular check-ups!), we are still working flat out with our legal team. Our daughter is home, but we will keep working on this important case – after all, we are here to make sure her future is safer and more prosperous.

Chapter 9

LESSONS LEARNED

UNCOMFORTABLE CONVERSATIONS: THE PRICE OF PROGRESS

The summer of 2016 is one I don't have many fond memories of. I was yearning for the freedom to test my wings, to carve a path that wasn't preordained by tradition. This disconnect created an uneasy feeling within me. It was a summer of wrestling with identities, of feeling like a stranger in my own skin and yearning for the day when the dissonance would fade.

I had just met a blogger online who wanted to write for my website, Feminism India, but was also keen on starting a podcast. After a few phone calls and planning, we decided to set up 'Desi Outsiders'. As a young girl in medical school, I suddenly felt myself tumbling into a divine mission. This podcast wouldn't just be about social media content; it would be a megaphone for silenced voices.

Launching Desi Outsiders made me feel like Joan of Arc, poised to lead a feminist charge with my virtual microphone. Yet my parents remained stubbornly entrenched in their traditional mindset and the very notion of my voice, unfiltered and raw, soaring through the internet, horrified them.

I had been trapped in a small box my whole life. This was the 'good Indian girl' my parents envisioned. Exploration, a life beyond the expected path, terrified them. It wasn't until medical school that I realised how dangerous this was. It wasn't just my parents who had clipped my wings – I realised that I, too, had unknowingly participated in my own confinement.

The playground taunts, the subtle stings of racism, they must have brushed past me unnoticed. Unlike the other children of colour in other parts of the world, I didn't carry the weight or the scars of those experiences. I always envisioned a world where opportunities wouldn't be coloured by the shade of my skin, a world where dreams wouldn't be dimmed by the weight of someone else's prejudice. It was a beautiful, yet tragically fragile, illusion.

As I grew older and started medical school, reality began to seep into the cracks of my sheltered world. The casual microaggressions, the sudden, suspicious glances in stores, the unspoken biases – they chipped away at the foundation of my innocent belief. The world wasn't quite as fair or meritocratic as I had once thought. A bittersweet realisation dawned – the path wouldn't be as smooth as I had imagined, and the fight for equality, a fight I hadn't even known I needed to be part of, would become a constant companion.

Decades of unspoken stories, unhealed wounds and unfulfilled dreams pressed down on my shoulders, a burden invisible to the eyes of those born into more privileged communities, who may never fully grasp the weight I carry. My race wasn't a sprint to the finish line, but a marathon fuelled by a desperate need to rewrite the narrative. Unlike many of my school friends, I wasn't just running for myself, but for the women who came before me, their yearning for education and opportunity echoing in my every step.

Prior to my protest, I would spend hours on the phone with my parents; I would even lose my voice trying to explain why this was so important to me. Some calls took us late into the middle of the night and I ended up in tears on numerous occasions. Every single day I would question myself and ask why I was putting myself under so much pressure to bring my parents on to my side. Was it really worth the tears and arguments?

I knew that their beliefs wouldn't change overnight and would swing back and forth like a pendulum. But the other option was to simply cut out the noise and forge my own path. Personally, that didn't feel right to me. Creating change means doing the work at home first, so that you can take your fight outside the walls of your house. It's very easy to have a group of people on your side and have them cheer you on if their values already align with your own.

But creating change is about inviting these difficult conversations and having these late-night conversations with your loved ones as it plants that seed of thought for them to ultimately make their own decision.

In the aftermath of the protest, social media buzzed with praise. Every 'like' and retweet on Twitter felt like a warm hand on my back, a wave of virtual solidarity drowning all of my doubts. It was tempting to ride this wave of validation, to let it fuel my every step. But a sobering truth lurked beneath the surface. The real world, with its entrenched beliefs and opposing voices, would still be there tomorrow, and the day after that.

Over the last few years, this has been where I have placed

a lot of my time and energy: engaging in conversations with anybody who disagrees with me rather than with those who cheer me along. A single mind, shifted ever so slightly, can ripple outwards, changing the course of conversations, influencing actions and shaping the world for generations to come. It's a slow, arduous process. But the potential harvest, the possibility of a future where understanding blooms instead of division, that's what keeps me going. It's exhausting, yes, but the echoes of a brighter tomorrow are a far more potent motivator than the fleeting comfort of agreement.

* * *

Every Thursday, throughout the first few months of the pandemic, the British public would stand on their doorsteps and clap for one minute to thank NHS and key workers. At first, it gave me a warm feeling and on the first Thursday, I remember tearing up. It gave me a boost of motivation and encouragement especially when we were dealing with so many unknowns. My neighbours at the time were both social workers and, along with their kids, they would bring out all their pots and pans to bang them to show their love and appreciation. Some neighbours had gone to the effort of redesigning their front garden with the colours of the NHS and displaying artwork made by their young children or grandchildren.

On one hand, we had the public roaring their support and love for us and on the other, our leaders with all the power to make a positive change, sitting back and watching. To make things worse, our politicians would stand outside the doors of Number 10 and parliament and clap every Thursday.

For a long time, I wondered why and how we allowed the

British public to fund and fuel the morale of NHS workers. It wasn't their job. Leaders had shrugged this responsibility off. As the Clap for Carers movement grew, many people started to question its purpose. The founder of the movement, Annemarie Plas, decided to call it off. After nine weeks of the country clanking their saucepans, illuminating buildings in blue and millions of people applauding on their doorsteps, many felt this movement was becoming politicised.

Politicians were posting videos of themselves on fancy rooftops in London applauding for NHS workers. Matt Hancock, the Health Secretary at the time, posted a video saying, 'A huge thank you to our incredible NHS and social care staff. We can never thank you enough for all that you are doing for the nation.'

There were numerous other occasions where politicians came on the media to express their gratitude for NHS workers. It felt like being stabbed in the back with a knife. When they clapped, it felt as if they were twisting the same knife they had stabbed us in the back with in the first place.

Once again, I had the same feeling in my stomach as I did in April 2020. Watching the Clap for Carers movement become co-opted by politicians made me very uncomfortable. This time around, however, things were slightly different. I was joined by a group of a few more brave doctors who wanted to go out and protest against this movement. After two short months, the adrenaline rush of the first protest had barely faded, and we were already plotting our second. We had the help of an incredible team of creatives at The Citizens, a not-for-profit organisation founded and led by Carole Cadwalladr. Throughout the pandemic, Carole stayed in touch with us and her adventurous nature was always itching to create more noise and heighten the voices of doctors – she helped us plan and execute this next protest.

Again, with this protest, I spent a lot of time discussing with Nishant how we could have the most impact through the imagery and our messaging. This was the last 'Clap' – a poignant farewell to a movement that had papered over cracks in the system. We decided to kneel on one knee as a sign of respect for our colleagues who had died.

We decided to do it on the last Clap for Carers, right outside 10 Downing Street, to emphasise the stark contrast between the lives of our politicians and the lives of NHS workers. Whitehall was flooded with cameras that evening for the last Clap for Carers, and it was clear that many of the news channels were very interested in what we were doing.

We stayed on one knee for the whole minute and right behind us, Boris Johnson came out in front of the cameras and clapped, loud and proud. He obviously turned his back and hurried back inside to his office after his photo opportunity. But we had to go back into our hospitals and face a different reality.

As predicted, this protest became very popular online.

One journalist had followed us through the streets of London and was live tweeting our protest. He caught us from the beginning and as we were dressed in scrubs and carrying placards, he sensed something interesting was about to happen. I obviously had no idea about this, but Nishant, who was working at the time, was following his live tweets and noticed one thing: many people took offence at the fact that we went down on one knee. Accusations of appropriation, of hijacking a movement not our own, poisoned the discourse. People of colour felt we'd trampled on their struggle. We intended it to be a gesture of respect but had inadvertently stirred a different kind of storm.

As with my previous protest, the support and the hundreds of positive reactions were overwhelming. The echo chamber of 'good jobs' and 'well saids' was familiar, a comforting warmth. But there were also voices laced with hurt, accusing us of borrowing a symbol without understanding its weight.

I felt I had a responsibility to engage with these voices and understand why they felt disrespected. It wasn't about winning an argument, but about learning a crucial lesson. The fight for justice, I realised, wasn't a solo act, but a delicate tapestry woven from countless threads. We'd snagged a strand belonging to another struggle, and now we had to mend it with empathy and understanding. This wasn't about ego or blind defence, but about becoming better allies and better listeners in the ongoing fight for a more equitable world.

The seeds of activism, I believe, are first sown not on picket lines or in protest marches, but at your dinner table at home. It's in the crucible of difficult conversations with family, navigating the minefield of ingrained ideologies, where true empathy is forged. This is how we learn to hold space for reflection.

Amid the online negativity, you can find genuine voices, those tinged with confusion and hurt. These are the ones who deserve our attention, the ones worth engaging with, even if it's a dance on eggshells. These are the voices we should listen to, the ones that resonate not with malice, but with confusion and hurt.

It's a delicate art, this engagement. Not all conversations will end in epiphanies or apologies. But for the few that do, the rewards are immense. After all, the most fertile ground for change isn't the anonymous wasteland of the internet, but the soil of human connection, nurtured by patience and a willingness to listen.

The first tweet that caught my eye was from a black doctor on Twitter who had tweeted that although he supports our message, he felt deeply uncomfortable that we knelt on one knee to protest.

At first, I felt upset and deflated. We were working so hard to help people just like him – doctors from ethnic minority groups were being disproportionately affected by the virus and we wanted to advocate for them. Maybe the one-knee gesture, a symbol of respect in our minds, had resonated with a different, more painful history in his.

This wasn't about winning him over. It was about acknowledging the complexity, the tangled web of lived experiences that impacted our perceptions. So, I decided to send him a message on Twitter and very calmly explained that this was never meant to offend anybody, but I was more than happy to have a Zoom call and discuss my thoughts behind this protest and why we took the decision to go on one knee. A thousand scenarios played out – a raging storm of anger, or a calm, measured response. Yet, the potential for understanding, for a sliver of progress, outweighed the fear. It was time to step outside the echo chamber, to meet discomfort head on, one uncomfortable conversation at a time.

We had a Zoom call the next day, just two days after the protest. It was a Saturday afternoon and Nishant had a day off, so I asked him to sit close by just for moral support. Nishant believed in having these conversations as much as I did. In fact, he encouraged me to send him a direct message. When we started the call, I began to track back to everything I had learned in medical school about communication skills, especially everything we had learned about empathy. I wanted to empathise with him and understand how he must have felt when he saw our protest. It took some inner work and deep reflection but I went into this conversation asking him: How can I be better? What mistakes did I make and how can I avoid that in the future?

I took on that personal responsibility and made myself uncomfortable. We explored why going on one knee may have felt offensive to some communities.

Former San Francisco 49ers quarterback Colin Kaepernick first protested against racial injustice and police brutality by kneeling down during the United States national anthem in the summer of 2016. Since then, a whole movement has grown up around that gesture. When I spoke to this doctor, we weren't aware at the time but going down on one knee would become a widespread theme in sport after the death of George Floyd in the United States.

The issue was clear: people felt that I had co-opted a gesture for my own political gain. Some were saying that it was 'tone deaf' and I understood why people felt this way considering all the trauma and mistreatment black communities were facing, especially in the United States. The symbol of taking the knee was a message of respect to the innocent black people who lost their lives in the hands of police brutality. The answer, then, wasn't in forcing a singular meaning onto the symbol. It was in understanding the kaleidoscope of perspectives.

As we explored my reasoning, I also invited this doctor to explain his own feelings and, ultimately, create a comfortable, open space for a discussion where we could both leave feeling that we had learned something new. I was reminded on a deeper level that we all have some form of privilege. As people of colour, we are not given the upper hand in society, but as a doctor I have certain privileges. As an educated woman, I have knowledge. I can never forget that. Although collectively, we are groups of people who are marginalised, within these bubbles, we must appreciate that there are different levels of privilege we all have, and understanding that is the key to helping others around us.

We explored the reasoning behind the gesture, the respect it was meant to convey. But more importantly, I created space for him to unveil his own experience. As we delved into the 'why' behind the protest and the 'why' behind his discomfort, a fragile bridge began to form. It wouldn't be a one-way street. My aim wasn't to convert him, but to create a space where understanding could bloom.

Being a doctor granted me a certain respect, an education that opened doors. Being a woman of colour meant navigating a different set of challenges. We were both marginalised, yet within those margins, invisible hierarchies existed. Recognising those hierarchies, and acknowledging them, was the key to unlocking empathy.

We had no qualms with each other by the end of the call. Perhaps, in this shared purpose, a new symbol could be forged, one of mutual respect.

BEYOND ACTIVISM: THE PERSONAL COST

During my time at home before giving birth, I worked on audit papers and, in between, answered calls from journalists and worried relatives – mainly my parents. I had no sense of time. Since I was at home, the days seemed endless. I could sleep when I wanted; I had no urgent commitments to wake up to and I could sit in bed with my laptop and do all my work. The only time I ventured outside was for my midwife appointments.

I had nothing to look forward to and nobody to meet up with and I constantly played scenarios in my head of how I would be able to give birth in a pandemic. Death, a grim companion on the wards, became a constant, unwelcome guest in my thoughts. It wasn't just me talking about the pandemic; the whole world was. The pandemic wasn't just a news story; it was the suffocating air we all breathed, stealing the joy from anticipation and replacing it with a gnawing dread.

Without realising, I soon started to feel the weight of this huge responsibility that I had taken on. It settled on me like a leaden cloak. Each day, it grew heavier. The exhaustion wasn't physical, but a deeper weariness of my soul. I was tired of the endless justifications, the constant need to prove the worth of my story to journalists. All I yearned for was the quiet solace of a corner, a reprieve from the constant performance of my bravery.

The life blooming within me should have been a vibrant ember, igniting a joyous fire of anticipation. But the relentless news and the weight of my decision had doused the flame. My tank, once overflowing with excitement, ran on fumes. Now, the ache of missed moments pierces me. Where was the thrill to build my baby's nursery? Where was the excitement to phone relatives and discuss baby names?

I wish I could rewind, to reclaim those stolen moments of joy, to replace the lonely darkness with the warm glow of anticipation.

When I had scheduled calls with our journalists, I'd cry myself to sleep the night before out of fear. I was terrified of looking and sounding like a fool. I felt that I didn't deserve to be in this position, to be leading a movement. So many people around me kept telling me that I wasn't doing the right thing and I was crazy for taking on such a big fight. I internalised these comments and they manifested in some very ugly ways. I would doubt myself and think twice before saying anything on important calls. On my bad days, I would use the excuse of my pregnancy to get out of phone calls because, at times, it all just became too much. Sometimes, the fight simply became too much to bear alone. In the quiet of those darkened days, curled under the duvet, I waged a different kind of battle – a desperate war against the voice that whispered, 'You're not good enough.'

The fire that had ignited my first protest had dwindled, replaced by a suffocating fog of doubt. Each night, as I drifted off to sleep, the fear of failure played on repeat – a haunting melody that stole the joy from my days. The world outside continued to fight the pandemic, but the battle I waged was now an internal one – a desperate struggle against the poisonous seeds I had unwittingly allowed to take root.

Social media, initially a wellspring of inspiration, morphed into a hall of mirrors reflecting distorted realities. Influencers and campaigners, their faces polished and their lives curated, seemed to exist on a different plane – a plane of effortless success. I asked myself, 'What does it mean to "make it" as an activist?' Social media can paint an idealistic belief that there is a finish line, a point where societal ills are vanquished. But progress is a relentless climb, not a summit to be conquered. There will always be another mountain to scale, another injustice to fight.

Maybe activism is a lifelong journey, a constant dance with ever-evolving societal issues. There will always be another mountain to climb, another injustice to fight. The 'making it' isn't about some external validation; it is about the unwavering belief that even the smallest voice can nudge the world in a better direction.

I lived with this big grey cloud hanging over my head for months. I had plenty of excuses to pull the plug, but I kept going. I knew that if I looked back at this time in ten years, regret would be a bitter pill to swallow.

To this day, I have had no contact with some of my family members. My beautiful daughters, with their infectious giggles and eyes that hold galaxies, are strangers to some who share my blood.

Yet, amid the wreckage of these fractured bonds, a tiny ember of defiance refuses to be extinguished. The fight for what I believed in, the fight for a better me, may have come at a heart-wrenching cost, but the alternative – staying silent – is an even more unbearable thought. For now, I carry the weight of this loss, a constant reminder of the price we sometimes pay for the courage to stand up and be heard.

Within the ache, a new-found strength takes root. The courage to be true to myself has forged a resilience within me. It's a resilience that whispers, 'This pain may shape you, but it will not break you. It will lead you to a place of greater strength, a place where your truth resonates not just within yourself, but in the symphony of the world.'

Chapter 10

NURTURING PURPOSE

Finding Joy and Fulfillment in Motherhood and Activism

Once, I floated on a cloud of idealism; a pregnant woman adrift in a world painted with pastel hues. I was free from the earthly tether of childcare, and financial burdens seemed a distant thunder. I found purpose and expressed myself through the digital and online world; it kept me going every single day. During a time where we were all isolated from our loved ones, I was in desperate search for warmth, a yearning for connection. Those digital bonds became my sunrise, the reason to face another day in my solitary abyss created by the pandemic. But the birth of my daughters was a cosmic shift, a tectonic plate rearranging my world. The once-crisp idealism blurred and was replaced by a raw, gritty reality. The gentle lullaby of expectation was drowned out by the urgent cries of the newborn.

With each tiny hand that curled around my finger, a piece of my former life slipped away. I thrived on intellectual stimulation, and the loss of social validation left me mourning for the person I once was. The transition from carefully crafting my online presence to the relentless rhythm of nappy changes was a bitter pill to swallow.

I felt that all the knowledge and experience I had gained was rotting away and there was nothing I could do about it. After all, I had a tiny baby who depended on me for everything. Slowly, as the months went on, I found pockets of peace during my day to sit down and continue the work I loved so much.

Apart from the gruelling routine of raising a newborn baby, I underestimated the impact of sleep deprivation and all the hormonal changes my body was going through. Sleep, once a comforting harbour, now became a distant mirage. My body betrayed me with a hormonal maelstrom, leaving me adrift in a sea of tears at the slightest provocation. The world outside, once filled with purpose, shrank to a mere whisper as I grappled with the weight of exhaustion.

I vividly recall a day that felt like an eternity as I tried to coax Radhika into sleep. The pressure of an impending article deadline weighed heavily on me that day, but all I could think about was getting her to nap, just for a little while. I walked endless laps around the neighbourhood, her tiny body nestled in the pram, and finally, after what felt like a marathon, she drifted into a peaceful sleep.

Relieved, I tiptoed back home, gently placed her down and rushed to plug in my laptop, ready to dive into my work. But just as the screen flickered to life, I heard it – the unmistakable wail that shattered the fragile silence. Radhika was awake, crying out with all her might, needing nothing more than to be held close. My deadline slipped further out of reach, and in that moment, all I could do was surrender to the reality that her need for comfort was far greater than my need to write.

Life has a way of surprising us, pulling us in directions we hadn't planned for. Just when we feel that we've found our purpose, life may intervene; perhaps a loved one falls ill, or our children need more of our time and love. In those moments, it's easy to feel that we're being pulled away from the path we've chosen, that we're losing precious time that could be spent fighting for the causes we believe in.

But here's the truth: there is no shame in stepping back. We are human, after all, with emotional needs and personal responsibilities that sometimes take precedence. It's important to remember that taking time for ourselves and our families doesn't mean we're abandoning our purpose. Rather, it's an essential part of sustaining the energy and compassion that fuel our activism.

In a world where social media constantly pressures us to be visible, to speak out without pause, we must ask ourselves: is it worth it if we're sacrificing our well-being and our ability to be present for those who matter most?

True activism isn't about the relentless pursuit of a cause at the expense of our own humanity. It's about finding balance, acknowledging when we need to pause and recharge, and understanding that caring for ourselves and our loved ones is just as important as the work we do in the world.

The intersection of activism and motherhood has been a powerful endeavour, as both roles require deep emotional investment and constant balancing. Although these are not always applicable, here are a few actionable tips that have worked for me during the last few years.

Spoiler alert: it won't always work, but if you use this as a general framework, I'm sure it will ease the burden we all feel to show up for our purpose and passion every single day.

1. SET BOUNDARIES AND PRIORITISE SELF-CARE

Establish clear boundaries between your activism work and your personal life. Allocate specific time slots for activism and family, ensuring that neither consumes all your energy.

For example, dedicate mornings to your activism efforts and reserve evenings for family time. During your family time, disconnect from work emails and social media to be fully present.

I would always try and work on my laptop when Radhika was taking a nap. Sometimes it was difficult knowing that there were dishes and laundry waiting to be tackled, but I had to learn to accept that some things just had to wait. (I still struggle with this; in fact, as I write this sentence, I have a sink full of dishes waiting to be washed.)

2. BUILD A SUPPORT NETWORK

Surround yourself with a community of like-minded individuals who understand the challenges of balancing motherhood and activism. This could include fellow activist mothers, supportive friends, or even online communities. If you're not a mother but have other caring responsibilities – such as looking after elderly parents, supporting a partner or caring for siblings or other dependents – seek out networks that share your unique experiences. These connections can provide both emotional support and practical advice, helping you navigate the delicate balance between caregiving and creating meaningful change in society.

Finding a space where you can vent, celebrate victories and gain perspective is priceless. Back then, I didn't have many friends who truly understood the passion driving me, and that loneliness weighed heavily on me. I'll never forget the day I sat there, scrolling through my Instagram feed, feeling the emptiness of those connections that didn't resonate with the fire I was trying so hard to keep alive. With each unfollow, it was as if I was shedding layers of what no longer served me, desperately trying to protect the fragile spark that fuelled my purpose.

3. EMBRACE IMPERFECTION AND FLEXIBILITY

It took me a while to understand that perfection is not the goal – it's about trusting the process. Allow yourself the grace to be imperfect and adapt to changes as they come.

If a planned event conflicts with a family obligation, it's okay to reschedule or modify your involvement. Similarly, on days when your emotional energy is low, focus on smaller, manageable tasks rather than pushing yourself too hard. Learning to let go and adapt has allowed me to become a better mother and activist and, most importantly, I've learned to forgive myself for my imperfections.

4. INCORPORATE MOMENTS OF JOY AND REST

Actively seek out and prioritise moments of joy and rest. There will be moments when you're so exhausted that even enjoying time with your children feels like a distant dream – I've been there more times than I can count! But showing up for them, for your family, is just as vital as any work deadline. These relationships are fragile and need your full attention and love, even if it means swapping your laptop for a tea party with your daughter's dolls, tucking them in on the sofa instead of tackling your to-do list. You might feel a twinge of guilt, but those precious moments are just as important as anything else you're working on.

Balancing activism and motherhood is a challenging but deeply fulfilling journey. By managing your emotional needs with intention and care, you can sustain your efforts and continue making a difference, both in the world and at home.

As you close this book, know that the journey of motherhood and activism is one of profound courage, love and resilience. You hold within you the power to nurture life and ignite change, to cradle the future while shaping the present. The road ahead may be challenging, but remember that every step you take, every voice you raise, and every act of kindness and protest, contributes to the world you want your children to inherit. Your passion is your guide, and your love is your strength. Together, they are unstoppable forces for good.

During my book writing process, I specifically made time to exercise and play the sports I love. Of course, there were times when I thought that perhaps I should be working on my writing instead of spending time at the gym, but forcing myself to take regular breaks allowed me to truly be present and enjoy working on this book.

So, as you go forward, let your heart lead the way. Embrace the moments of joy and the trials that come with this dual path. Stand tall in your truth, knowing that your actions, however small, ripple out into the world, creating waves of change. This is your call to action: to live fully, love fiercely and fight boldly for the things that matter most. You are not just a mother, not just an activist – you are a beacon of hope, lighting the way for those who will follow. The world needs your voice, your passion, your strength, now more than ever. So go out there and make the difference only you can make.

Endnotes

Chapter 1

1 Rizan, C., Reed, M. & Bhutta, M.F. (2021) Environmental impact of personal protective equipment distributed for use by health and social care services in England in the first six months of the COVID-19 pandemic. *Journal of the Royal Society of Medicine*, 114(5), 250–263. https://journals.sagepub.com/doi/full/10.1177/01410768211001583.

2 BBC (2022) Covid-19: Government writes off £8.7bn of pandemic PPE. www.bbc.co.uk/news/uk-60176283.

3 Public Health England (2017) Exercise Cygnus Report. https://assets.publishing.service.gov.uk/government/uploads/system/uploads/attachment_data/file/927770/exercise-cygnus-report.pdf.

4 Department of Health and Social Care (2020) UK pandemic preparedness. www.gov.uk/government/publications/uk-pandemic-preparedness.

5 Heffer, G. (2020, 22 March) Coronavirus: NHS staff urge PM to provide more protective equipment as two consultants receive critical care. Sky News. https://news.sky.com/story/coronavirus-nhs-staff-urge-pm-to-provide-more-protective-equipment-as-two-consultants-receive-critical-care-11961900.

Chapter 3

1 Royal College of Obstetricians and Gynaecologists (2020) Coronavirus (COVID-19) infection in pregnancy: information for healthcare professionals. Version 2: published Friday 13 March 2020. www.readkong.com/page/coronavirus-covid-19-infection-in-pregnancy-5792039.

2 Cvorak, M. (2020, 20 March) 'Coronavirus has hospitals on a war footing': A&E doctor calls for urgent help – video. *The Guardian*. www.theguardian.com/world/video/2020/mar/20/coronavirus-has-hospitals-on-a-war-footing-ae-doctor-calls-for-urgent-help-video.

3 Cadwalladr, C. (2020, 16 March) 'Everyone is scared to speak up': A&E doctor asks for Covid-19 tests. *The Guardian*. www.theguardian.com/world/2020/mar/16/everyone-is-scared-to-speak-up-nhs-staff-need-covid-19-tests.

4 Sahib, B. (2020, 23 April) Legal challenge against the UK government's guidance about personal protective equipment in hospitals. Bindmans. www.bindmans.com/news-insights/news/legal-challenge-against-the-uk-governments-guidance-about-personal-protective-equipment-in-hospitals.

5 Booth, R. (2020, 19 March) Temporary morgues being set up across UK amid rising Covid-19 deaths. *The Guardian*. www.theguardian.com/world/2020/mar/19/temporary-morgues-being-set-up-across-uk-amid-rising-covid-19-deaths.

6 Campbell, D. (2020, 31 March) NHS staff 'gagged' over coronavirus shortages. *The Guardian*. www.theguardian.com/society/2020/mar/31/nhs-staff-gagged-over-coronavirus-protective-equipment-shortages.

7 Francis, R. (2013) *Report of the Mid Staffordshire NHS Foundation Trust Public Inquiry*. The Stationery Office. https://assets.publishing.service.gov.uk/media/5a7ba0faed915d13110607c8/0947.pdf?.

8 Francis, R. (2013) *Report of the Mid Staffordshire NHS Foundation Trust Public Inquiry*. The Stationery Office. https://assets.publishing.service.gov.uk/media/5a7ba0faed915d13110607c8/0947.pdf?.

9 Francis, R. (2015) *Freedom to Speak Up Report*. Department of Health. www.freedomtospeakup.org.uk/wp-content/uploads/2014/07/F2SU_web.pdf.

Chapter 4

1 Nie, J.B. & Elliott, C. (2020) Humiliating whistle-blowers: Li Wenliang, the response to Covid-19, and the call for a decent society. *Journal of Bioethical Inquiry*, 17(4), 543–547. https://pmc.ncbi.nlm.nih.gov/articles/PMC7445730.

Chapter 7

1 Marsh, S. (2020, 20 April) At least 100 UK health workers have died from coronavirus, figures show. *The Guardian*. www.theguardian.com/world/2020/apr/20/at-least-100-uk-health-workers-have-died-from-coronavirus-figures-show.

Chapter 8

1 Bowcott, O. (2020, 24 April) Doctor couple challenge UK government on PPE risks to BAME staff. *The Guardian*. www.theguardian.com/world/2020/apr/24/doctor-couple-challenge-uk-government-on-ppe-risks-to-bame-staff.

2 Reuters (2020, 23 April) Doctors launch legal challenge to UK government over protective kit. www.reuters.com/article/us-health-coronavirus-britain-legal/doctors-launch-legal-challenge-to-uk-government-over-protective-kit-idUSKCN22533P.

3 Campbell, D. (2020, 23 April) Emails reveal doctor's plea for PPE before Covid-19 death. *The Guardian*. www.theguardian.com/society/2020/apr/23/emails-reveal-doctors-plea-for-ppe-before-covid-19-death-dr-peter-tun.

4 Gov.uk (2020, 10 January) COVID-19: infection prevention and control (IPC). www.gov.uk/government/publications/wuhan-novel-coronavirus-infection-prevention-and-control.

5 Cook, T., Kursumovic, E. & Lennane, S. (2020, 22 April) Exclusive: deaths of NHS staff from covid-19 analysed. HSJ. www.hsj.co.uk/exclusive-deaths-of-nhs-staff-from-covid-19-analysed/7027471.article.

6 BBC (2020, 22 April) Coronavirus: Government facing fresh questions over EU equipment scheme. www.bbc.com/news/uk-politics-52377087.amp.

7 The Faculty of Intensive Care Medicine, Intensive Care Society and Association of Anaesthetists (2020, 19 April) Joint statement from UK anaesthetic and intensive care bodies in response to updated PPE guidance. https://icmanaesthesiacovid-19.org/news/joint-statement-from-uk-anaesthetic-and-intensive-care-bodies-in-response-to-updated-ppe-guidance.

8 Smedley, S. (2020, 21 April) Ministers face anger at PPE shortage for NHS staff. *News and Star* www.newsandstar.co.uk/news/18393317.ministers-face-anger-ppe-shortage-nhs-staff.

9 Nie, J.B. & Elliott, C. (2020) Humiliating whistle-blowers: Li Wenliang, the response to Covid-19, and the call for a decent society. *Journal of Bioethical Inquiry*, 17(4), 543–547. https://pmc.ncbi.nlm.nih.gov/articles/PMC7445730.

10 Cadwalladr, C. (2020, 16 March) 'Everyone is scared to speak up': A&E doctor asks for Covid-19 tests. *The Guardian*. www.theguardian.com/world/2020/mar/16/everyone-is-scared-to-speak-up-nhs-staff-need-covid-19-tests.

11 Hartley-Parkinson, R. (2020, 16 April) Fundraiser for baby of pregnant nurse who died from coronavirus heads towards £100,000. Metro. https://metro.co.uk/2020/04/16/fundraiser-baby-pregnant-nurse-died-coronavirus-heads-towards-100000-12563402.

12 BBC News (2020, 24 April) Coronavirus: doctors launch legal challenge over PPE guidance. www.bbc.co.uk/news/uk-england-beds-bucks-herts-52411814.

13 Cadwalladr, C. (2020, 20 April) 'They can't get away with this': doctor who took protest to No 10. *The Guardian*. www.theguardian.com/society/2020/apr/20/coronavirus-doctor-ppe-protest-downing-street-london.

14 Shepherd, A. (2020, 2 June) Covid-19: frontline doctors continue PPE fight. *BMJ*. www.bmj.com/content/369/bmj.m2188.

15 Viz, M. & Joshi, N. (2020, 4 June) The government's reaction to BAME deaths tells us everything we already knew about our society. Byline Times. https://bylinetimes.com/2020/06/04/the-governments-reaction-to-bame-deaths-tells-us-everything-we-already-knew-about-our-society/?fbclid=IwAR1MA5CU9QvNgM-iZxJtZ4e7t1nf0kG4dXi57C0E8QKCxIU9Eiw2Oxyk3wM.